Errors in Veterinary Anesthesia

T0317623

Errors in Veterinary Anesthesia

John W. Ludders, DVM, DipACVAA

Professor Emeritus, College of Veterinary Medicine,
Cornell University, Ithaca, NY, USA

Matthew McMillan, BVM&S, DipECVAA, MRCVS

Clinical Anaesthetist, Department of Veterinary Medicine,
University of Cambridge, Cambridge, UK

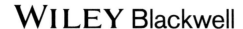

Editorial Offices

1606 Golden Aspen Drive, Suites 103 and 104, Ames, Iowa 50010, USA

The Atrium, Southern Gate, Chichester, West Sussex, PO19 8SQ, UK

9600 Garsington Road, Oxford, OX4 2DQ, UK

For details of our global editorial offices, for customer services and for information about how to apply for permission to reuse the copyright material in this book please see our website at www.wiley.com/wiley-blackwell.

Library of Congress Cataloging-in-Publication Data

Names: Ludders, John W., author. | McMillan, Matthew, author.
Title: Errors in veterinary anesthesia / John W. Ludders, Matthew McMillan.
Description: Ames, Iowa : John Wiley & Sons, Inc, 2017. | Includes bibliographical references and index.
Identifiers: LCCN 2016022481| ISBN 9781119259718 (cloth) | ISBN 9781119259732 (Adobe PDF) |
    ISBN 9781119259725 (epub)
Subjects: LCSH: Veterinary anesthesia. | Medical errors. | MESH: Medical Errors–veterinary |
    Anesthesia–veterinary | Medical Errors–prevention & control
Classification: LCC SF914 .L77 2017 | NLM SF 914 | DDC 636.089/796–dc23
LC record available at https://lccn.loc.gov/2016022481

A catalogue record for this book is available from the British Library.

Set in 8.5/12pt Meridien by SPi Global, Pondicherry, India

1   2017

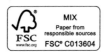

To veterinary anesthetists who err and wonder why

Contents

Preface

It's a busy night of emergencies. A puppy, having eaten its owner's socks, is undergoing exploratory abdominal surgery for gastrointestinal obstruction. A young tomcat is being treated for urinary tract obstruction, and a Pomeranian with a prolapsed eye has just been admitted as has a dog with multiple lacerations from a dog fight. A German shepherd with gastric dilatation and volvulus is being treated in one of the two bays in the emergency treatment room. This evening is also a new employee's first night on duty; she and two other staff members are assisting with the German shepherd dog. After initially stabilizing the dog, it is anesthetized with fentanyl and propofol and then intubated so as to facilitate passing a stomach tube to decompress its stomach. The new employee, who is unfamiliar with the emergency practice's standard operating procedures, facilities, and equipment, is told to attach an oxygen insufflation hose to the endotracheal tube. The employee inserts the hose into the endotracheal tube rather than attach it to a flow-by device, a device that is small and located out of sight at the other treatment bay. By inserting the insufflation hose into the endotracheal tube the patient's airway is partially obstructed; the oxygen flow is set at $5\,L\,min^{-1}$ (Figure 1). No one notices the error because the rest of the team is focused on inserting the stomach tube; within a few minutes the dog has a cardiac arrest. During CPR, which is ultimately unsuccessful, the team recognizes that the dog has a pneumothorax and its source is quickly identified.

Why do well-trained and caring professionals make errors such as this? How should the veterinarian in charge of the emergency respond to this accident? How can a veterinarian or practice anticipate an error or accident such as this so that it can be avoided, or prevented from occurring again? Both of us have thought about and explored the hows and whys of

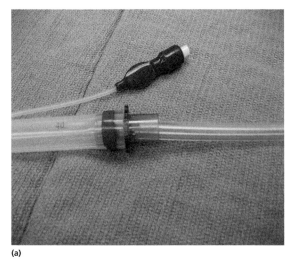

(a)

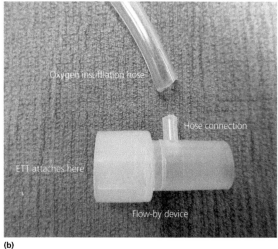

(b)

Figure 1 **a)** Insufflation hose inserted into an endotracheal tube almost completely occluding it. **b)** Flow-by device with connector where the oxygen insufflation hose is supposed to attach. The flow-by device is nothing more than an endotracheal tube (ETT) adaptor with a connector normally used with a gas analyzer for sampling and analyzing airway gases from an anesthetized, intubated animal. Using it for insufflating oxygen is a unique application of this device, not a usual one, and probably not a familiar one for the new employee of this practice.

errors that occur during anesthesia. Based on our experiences and as teachers of anesthesia to veterinary students and residents, it is our opinion that the answers lie in the reality that we can and must learn from errors; they are learning opportunities, not personal or professional stigmata highlighting our failings for all to see. How those of us involved in veterinary medicine, specifically those of us in doing and teaching veterinary anesthesia, can learn from errors is the purpose of this text.

John W. Ludders
Matthew McMillan

Acknowledgments

We cannot thank enough those who have supported and encouraged us in the writing of this book. A number of colleagues kindly read various drafts of this book, and their comments helped us clarify initial thoughts as to how the topic of errors in veterinary anesthesia should be approached. Most important was their encouragement to push on with the writing.

Some colleagues expended a great deal of time in reviewing a first draft. Looking back at that draft makes us appreciate their efforts even more. Two individuals deserve special mention. Dr Erik Hofmeister at the University of Georgia, pointed out details we came to realize were not important to the subject matter; his comments were especially helpful in structuring and writing what is now Chapter 2. Dr Daniel Pang at the University of Calgary, made extensive comments throughout the draft, comments that encouraged us to do a better job of using terminology consistently, and to develop concepts more thoroughly and link them more effectively to the cases we have included.

When faced with questions about various concepts in patient safety, concepts that are evolving as this book was being written, we asked for advice from individuals who are experts in various aspects of this field. We were pleasantly surprised to find that these individual were approachable and willing to give of their time and share their knowledge. Dr Marjorie Steigler at the University of North Carolina-Chapel Hill and Director of the Consortium of Anesthesiology Patient Safety and Experiential Learning, provided references and her thoughts concerning issues relating to effective training strategies for residents. Dr Allisa Russ at the Roudebush Veterans Administration Medical Center and the Regenstrief Institute, and who is involved in developing processes for reducing medication errors, generously shared her knowledge about human factors analysis, what it is and what it is not.

John Wiley & Sons, our publisher, have also been very supportive since we first approached them. We were both surprised and thankful that the concept of writing a book about error in veterinary anesthesia, something we feared might have been perceived as too much of a niche subject, was accepted in such an enthusiastic manner.

Throughout the writing process our families have encouraged and assisted us in our efforts. In particular, our wives, Kathy (J.W.L.) and Sam (M.W.M.), have tolerated a huge amount of inconvenience and disruption of the routines of family life. Without their support, encouragement, and sacrifices this book would not have been possible. We are as always in their debt.

Finally, as with any book there will be errors and they are our errors alone, we are after all only human.

Introduction

Knowledge and error flow from the same mental sources, only success can tell the one from the other.

Ernst Mach, 1905

There are many veterinary anesthesia texts on how to anesthetize a variety of animal patients; such is not the purpose of this text. It does, however, have everything to do with the processes involved in anesthetizing animal patients, from pre-anesthetic assessment to recovery, and does so by seeking answers to how and why errors occur during anesthesia. In this text we define an error as a failure to carry out a planned action as intended (error of execution), or the use of an incorrect or inappropriate plan (error of planning), while an adverse incident is a situation where harm has occurred to a patient or a healthcare provider as a result of some action or event. How can those who are responsible for the anesthetic management of patients detect and manage unexpected errors and accidents during anesthesia? How can we learn from errors and accidents?

In the heat of the moment when a patient under our care suffers a life-threatening injury or dies, it is natural to look for something or someone to blame; usually the person who "made the mistake." This is a normal response. Subsequently we may reprimand and chastise the individual who caused the accident and, by so doing, assume we've identified the source of the problem and prevented it from ever occurring again. Unfortunately, such is not the case because this approach fails to take into account two realities: (1) all humans, without exception, make errors (Allnutt 1987); and (2) errors are often due to latent conditions within the organization, conditions that set the stage for the error or accident and that were present long before the person who erred was hired. We can either acknowledge these realities and take steps to learn from errors and accidents, or we can deny them, for whatever reasons, be they fear of criticism or litigation, and condemn ourselves to make the same or similar errors over and over again (Adams 2005; Allnutt 1987; Edmondson 2004; Leape 1994, 2002; Reason 2000, 2004; Woods 2005).

In general there are two approaches to studying and solving the problem of human fallibility and the making of errors: the person approach (also called proximate cause analysis) and the systems approach (Reason 2000). The person approach focuses on individuals and their errors, and blames them for forgetfulness, inattention, or moral weakness. This approach sees errors arising primarily from aberrant mental processes, such as forgetfulness, inattention, poor motivation, carelessness, negligence, and recklessness (Reason 2000). Those who follow this approach may use countermeasures such as poster campaigns that appeal to people's sense of fear, develop new procedures or add to existing ones, discipline the individual who made the error, threaten litigation, or name, blame, and shame the individual who erred (Reason 2000). It's an approach that tends to treat errors as moral issues because it assumes bad things happen to bad people—what psychologists call the "just world hypothesis" (Reason 2000).

In contrast, the systems approach recognizes the fundamental reality that humans always have and always will make errors, a reality we cannot change. But we can change the conditions under which people work so as to build defenses within the system, defenses designed to avert errors or mitigate their effects (Diller *et al.* 2014; Reason 2000; Russ *et al.* 2013). Proponents of the systems approach strive for a comprehensive error management program that considers the multitude of factors that lead to errors, including organizational, environmental, technological, and other system factors.

Some, however, have misgivings about these two approaches as means of preventing errors in medical practice. A prevalent view is that clinicians are personally responsible for ensuring the safe care of their patients and a systems or human factors analysis approach will lead clinicians to behave irresponsibly, that is, they will blame errors on the system and not take personal responsibility for their errors (Leape 2001). Dr Lucian Leape, an advocate of the systems approach, points out that these thoughts only perpetuate the culture of blame that permeates healthcare (Leape 2001). The essence of systems theory is that human errors are caused by system failures that can be prevented by redesigning work environments so that it is difficult or impossible to make errors that harm patients (Leape 2001). Leape contends that this approach does not lessen a clinician's responsibility, but deepens and broadens it; when an error does occur the clinician has a responsibility—an obligation—to future patients to ask how the error could have been prevented, thus questioning the system with all of its component parts. Leape goes on to say that fears about "blameless" medicine are unfounded and are related to the universal tendency to confuse the making of an error with misconduct (Leape 2001). Misconduct, the willful intent to mislead or cause harm, is never to be tolerated in healthcare. Multiple studies in many different types of environments including healthcare, have shown that the majority of errors—95% or more—are made by well-trained, well-meaning, conscientious people who are trying to do their job well, but who are caught in faulty systems that set them up to make mistakes and who become "second victims" (Leape 2001). People do not go to work with the intent of making errors or causing harm.

This text is written with a bias toward the systems approach, a bias that has grown out of our experiences as anesthetists, as teachers of anesthesia to veterinary students, residents, and technicians, and as individuals who believe in the principles and practices underlying continuous quality improvement. This latter stance is not unique and reflects a movement toward the systems approach in the larger world of healthcare (Chang et al. 2005).

No part of this book is written as a criticism of others. Far from it. Many of the errors described herein are our own or those for which we feel fully responsible. Our desire is to understand how and why we make errors in anesthesia so as to discover how they can be prevented, or more quickly recognized and managed. We believe that the systems approach allows us to do just that. It is also an approach that can be used to help teach the principles of good anesthetic management to those involved in veterinary anesthesia. This approach also has broader applicability to the larger world of veterinary medicine.

This text consists of eight chapters. The first chapter is divided into two sections, the first of which briefly discusses terminology and the use of terms within the domain of patient safety. The reader is strongly encouraged to read the brief section on terminology because it defines the terms we use throughout this book. Terms, in and of themselves, do not explain why or how errors occur; that is the purpose of the second section, which provides some answers to the "whys" and "hows" of error genesis. This discussion draws upon a large body of literature representing the results of studies into the causes and management of errors and accidents; a body of literature spanning the fields of psychology, human systems engineering, medicine, and the aviation, nuclear, and petrochemical industries. This section is not an exhaustive review of the literature, but is meant to acquaint the reader with error concepts and terminology that are the basis for understanding why and how errors happen.

Terminology, especially abbreviations, can be a source of error. In the medical literature many terms are abbreviated under the assumption they are so common that their meanings are fully recognized and understood by all readers. For example, ECG is the abbreviation for electrocardiogram unless, of course, you are accustomed to EKG, which derives from the German term. It is assumed that every reader know that "bpm" signifies "beats per minute" for heart rate. But wait a minute! Could that abbreviation be used for breaths per minute? Or, what about blood pressure monitoring? And therein is the problem. A number of studies have clearly shown that abbreviations, although their use is well intentioned and meant to reduce verbiage, can be confusing, and out of that confusion misunderstandings and errors arise (Brunetti 2007; Kilshaw et al. 2010; Parvaiz et al. 2008; Sinha et al. 2011). This reality has led us to avoid using abbreviations as much as possible throughout the book. In the few instances where we do use abbreviations, primarily in the chapters describing cases and near misses, we spell the terms in full and include in parentheses the abbreviations that will be used in that particular case or near miss vignette. It seems like such a minor detail in the realm of error prevention, but the devil is in the details.

The second chapter presents the multiple factors that cause errors, including organizational, supervisory, environmental, personnel, and individual factors. At the organizational level the discussion focuses on organizational features that are the hallmarks of "learning organizations" or "high reliability organizations," organizations with a culture attuned to error prevention and a willingness and ability to learn from errors. Because individuals are at the forefront—at the sharp end—of systems where errors occur this chapter discusses cognitive factors that can lead to error generation.

The third chapter focuses on strategies by which we can proactively deal with errors. To be proactive an individual or organization has to be knowledgeable about the environment within which work is performed and errors occur. This knowledge can only come from collecting and analyzing data about patient safety incidents. To act there have to be reporting systems in place that provide information that accurately reflects the working of the organization, including its culture, policies, and procedures, and, of course, the people who work within the organization. This chapter especially focuses on voluntary reporting systems and the key features that make such systems successful. Reporting an incident is critical, but so too is the process of analysis, and this chapter presents some strategies and techniques for analyzing errors and accidents. It does so by using a systems approach and presents concepts and techniques such as root cause analysis and Ishikawa diagrams (fishbone diagrams). This chapter also presents a process by which accountability for an error can be determined so as to distinguish between the healthcare provider who intentionally causes harm (misconduct) in contrast to the individual who is the unfortunate victim of a faulty system.

Chapters 4 through 7 present and discuss cases and near misses that have occurred in veterinary anesthesia. Each chapter has an error theme: Chapter 4 presents cases and near miss vignettes involving technical and equipment errors; Chapter 5 medication errors; Chapter 6 clinical decision-making and diagnostic errors, and Chapter 7 communication errors. After reading these chapters some readers may object to our classification scheme. Indeed, we created the chapters and grouped the cases and near misses according to our assessment of the final act/proximate cause of the error, not in terms of their root causes. Although this is contrary to the approach we advocate throughout the book for dealing with errors, it has enabled us to resolve two issues with which we had to contend while developing these chapters. Firstly, not all cases underwent a thorough analysis at the time they occurred, making it difficult to retrospectively establish with certainty the root causes of a number of the errors and near misses. Secondly, the themes of the chapters allow us to present cases and near misses that have common themes even though they may seem dissimilar because of the context in which they occurred.

Some of the cases involve patients that many veterinarians will never see in practice, such as the polar bear (see Case 6.1). Such unusual cases superficially may seem of limited value for understanding how errors occur. Although the error itself is unique (involving an exotic species or unfamiliar drug combinations), the many factors involved in the evolution of the incident have a high likelihood of occurring anywhere and with any patient regardless of species, anesthetics used, or procedures performed. We need to recognize the multitude of factors that predispose to making errors in any situation and also embrace the problem-solving processes that can be applied to manage them.

A word of caution to our readers: while reading these cases a natural response is to think, "What was the anesthetist thinking?!?! It's so obvious, why didn't the anesthetist see the problem?" In the retelling of these cases all too often clues are given that were not apparent at the time of the error. Indeed, these cases are retold with full use of the "retrospective scope," which, with its hindsight bias, influences how one perceives and judges the described events (see "Pattern-matching and biases" in Chapter 2, and Table 2.3). Remember, the view was not as clear to the anesthetist involved at the time of the error as it is in these pages.

The near miss vignettes represent errors that occur in veterinary anesthesia but do not cause patient harm only because the errors were caught and corrected early. These types of errors are also called "harmless hits" or "harmless incidents." Although we can learn a great deal from adverse incidents, such as the cases described in these four chapters, they are rare and the knowledge gained is often at the expense of a patient's well-being. Near misses, on the other hand, occur frequently and serve as indicators of problems or conditions within the system that have the potential to cause patient harm (Wu 2004).

The eighth and final chapter presents general and specific ideas and strategies for creating a patient safety organization, one in which patient safety as a cultural norm is paramount and permeates the organization. Training is an essential component of such a program. Throughout this chapter we present and discuss, in varying detail, some strategies and techniques that can be incorporated into training programs so that trainees have a proactive view of errors rather than a negative view (i.e., we all make errors, so let's learn from them), and are better prepared to identify and neutralize errors before they cause patient harm, or to mitigate their effects once identified.

The Appendices contain supplemental material supporting various concepts discussed in the book, such as guidelines and checklists.

This book is an introduction to error in veterinary anesthesia, it is not a definitive text on the subject. As such, we hope this book contributes to changing the perception that errors and mistakes happen only to bad or incompetent anesthetists or veterinarians, that it helps move the veterinary profession and the various regulatory agencies that monitor the profession, to recognize and accept that errors happen despite our best intentions and efforts. We need to move beyond the "name, blame, and shame" mentality and direct our energies at taking positive steps toward helping ourselves and others learn from our errors, fundamental steps that we can and must take if we are to reduce error and improve the safety of veterinary anesthesia. Our hope is that this book contributes to this journey.

References

Adams, H. (2005) 'Where there is error, may we bring truth.' A misquote by Margaret Thatcher as she entered No. 10, Downing Street in 1979. *Anaesthesia* **60**(3): 274–277.

Allnutt, M.F. (1987) Human factors in accidents. *British Journal of Anaesthesia* **59**(7): 856–864.

Brunetti, L. (2007) Abbreviations formally linked to medication errors. *Healthcare Benchmarks and Quality Improvement* **14**(11): 126–128.

Chang, A., *et al.* (2005) The JCAHO patient safety event taxonomy: A standardized terminology and classification schema for near misses and adverse events. *International Journal for Quality in Health Care* **17**(2): 95–105.

Diller, T., *et al.* (2014) The human factors analysis classification system (HFACS) applied to health care. *American Journal of Medical Quality* **29**(3): 181–190.

Edmondson, A.C. (2004) Learning from failure in health care: Frequent opportunities, pervasive barriers. *Quality & Safety in Health Care* **13**(Suppl. 2): ii3–9.

Kilshaw, M.J., *et al.* (2010) The use and abuse of abbreviations in orthopaedic literature. *Annals of the Royal College of Surgeons of England* **92**(3): 250–252.

Leape, L.L. (1994) Error in medicine. *Journal of the American Medical Association* **272**(23): 1851–1857.

Leape, L.L. (2001) Foreword: Preventing medical accidents: Is "systems analysis" the answer? *American Journal of Law & Medicine* **27**(2–3): 145–148.

Leape, L.L. (2002) Reporting of adverse events. *New England Journal of Medicine* **347**(20): 1633–1638.

Parvaiz, M.A., *et al.* (2008) The use of abbreviations in medical records in a multidisciplinary world–an imminent disaster. *Communication & Medicine* **5**(1): 25–33.

Reason, J.T. (2000) Human error: Models and management. *British Medical Journal* **320**(7237): 768–770.

Reason, J.T. (2004) Beyond the organisational accident: The need for "error wisdom" on the frontline. *Quality and Safety in Health Care* **13**(Suppl. 2): ii28–ii33.

Russ, A.L., *et al.* (2013) The science of human factors: Separating fact from fiction. *BMJ Quality & Safety* **22**(10): 802–808.

Sinha, S., *et al.* (2011) Use of abbreviations by healthcare professionals: What is the way forward? *Postgraduate Medical Journal* **87**(1029): 450–452.

Woods, I. (2005) Making errors: Admitting them and learning from them. *Anaesthesia* **60**(3): 215–217.

Wu, A.W. (2004) Is there an obligation to disclose near-misses in medical care? In: *Accountability – Patient Safety and Policy Reform* (ed. V.A. Sharpe). Washington, DC: Georgetown University Press, pp. 135–142.

CHAPTER 1

Errors: Terminology and Background

In effect, all animals are under stringent selection pressure to be as stupid as they can get away with.
  P.J. Richardson and R. Boyd in Not by genes alone: How culture transformed human evolution. University of Chicago Press, 2005.

The rule that human beings seem to follow is to engage the brain only when all else fails—and usually not even then.
  D.L. Hull in Science and selection: Essays on biological evolution and the philosophy of science. Cambridge University Press, 2001.

Error: terminology

Why read about taxonomy and terminology? They seem so boring and too "ivory tower." When starting to write this section, I (J.W.L.) recalled a warm September afternoon many years ago when I was a first-year veterinary student at Washington State University. It was in the anatomy lab that my lab partner and I were reading *Miller's Guide to the Dissection of the Dog* and thinking how we would rather be outside enjoying the lovely fall weather. At one point, my lab partner, now Dr Ron Wohrle, looked up and said, "I think I'm a fairly intelligent person, but I've just read this one sentence and I only understand three words: 'and,' 'the,' and 'of'." Learning anatomy was not only about the anatomy of the dog, cat, cow, and horse, it was also about learning the language of veterinary medicine.

Each profession or specialty has its own language—terminology—and the study of errors is no exception. Indeed, words and terms convey important concepts that, when organized into an agreed taxonomy, make it possible for those involved in all aspects of patient safety to communicate effectively across the broad spectrum of medicine. However, despite publication of the Institute of Medicine's report "To Err is Human" (Kohn *et al.* 2000) in 2000 and the subsequent publication of many articles and books concerning errors and patient safety, a single agreed taxonomy with its attendant terminology does not currently exist. This is understandable for there are many different ways to look at the origins of errors because there are many different settings within which

they occur, and different error classifications serve different needs (Reason 2005). But this shortcoming has made it difficult to standardize terminology and foster communication among patient safety advocates (Chang *et al.* 2005; Runciman *et al.* 2009). For example, the terms "near miss," "close call," and "preventable adverse event" have been used to describe the same concept or type of error (Runciman *et al.* 2009). Runciman reported that 17 definitions were found for "error" and 14 for "adverse event" while another review found 24 definitions for "error" and a range of opinions as to what constitutes an error (Runciman *et al.* 2009).

Throughout this book we use terms that have been broadly accepted in human medicine and made known globally through the World Health Organization (WHO 2009) and many publications, a few of which are cited here (Runciman *et al.* 2009; Sherman *et al.* 2009; Thomson *et al.* 2009). However, we have modified the terms used in physician-based medicine for use in veterinary medicine and have endeavored to reduce redundancy and confusion concerning the meaning and use of selected terms. For example, "adverse incident," "harmful incident," "harmful hit," and "accident" are terms that have been used to describe the same basic concept: a situation where patient harm has occurred as a result of some action or event; throughout this book we use a single term—"harmful incident"—to capture this specific concept. Box 1.1 contains selected terms used frequently throughout this text, but we strongly encourage the reader to review the list of terms and their definitions in Appendix B.

Errors in Veterinary Anesthesia, First Edition. John W. Ludders and Matthew McMillan.
© 2017 John Wiley & Sons, Inc. Published 2017 by John Wiley & Sons, Inc.

Box 1.1 Selected terms and definitions used frequently in this book.

Adverse incident An event that caused harm to a patient.

Adverse reaction Unexpected harm resulting from an appropriate action in which the correct process was followed within the context in which the incident occurred.

Error Failure to carry out a planned action as intended (error of execution), or use of an incorrect or inappropriate plan (error of planning).

Error of omission An error that occurs as a result of an action not taken. Errors of omission may or may not lead to adverse outcomes.

Harmful incident An incident that reached a patient and caused harm (harmful hit) such that there was a need for more or different medication, a longer stay in hospital, more tests or procedures, disability, or death.

Harmless incident An incident that reached a patient, but did not result in discernible harm (harmless hit).

Latent conditions Unintended conditions existing within a system or organization as a result of design, organizational attributes, training, or maintenance, and that lead to errors. These conditions often lie dormant in a system for lengthy periods of time before an incident occurs.

Mistake Occurs when a plan is inadequate to achieve its desired goal even though the actions may be appropriate and run according to plan; a mistake can occur at the planning stage of both rule-based and knowledge-based levels of performance.

Near miss An incident that for whatever reason, including by chance or timely intervention, did not reach the patient.

Negligence Failure to use such care as a reasonably prudent and careful person would use under similar circumstances.

Patient safety incident A healthcare-related incident or circumstance (situation or factor) that could have resulted, or did result, in unnecessary harm to a patient even if there is no permanent effect on the patient.

Risk The probability that an incident will occur.

Root cause analysis A systematic iterative process whereby the factors that contribute to an incident are identified by reconstructing the sequence of events and repeatedly asking "why?" until the underlying root causes have been elucidated.

System failure A fault, breakdown, or dysfunction within an organization or its practices, operational methods, processes, or infrastructure.

Veterinary healthcare-associated harm Impairment of structure or function of the body due to plans or actions taken during the provision of healthcare, rather than as a result of an underlying disease or injury; includes disease, injury, suffering, disability, and death.

Terminology in and of itself, however, does not explain how errors occur. For that we need to look at models and concepts that explain the generation of errors in anesthesia.

Error: background

The model often used to describe the performance of an anesthetist is that of an airplane pilot; both are highly trained and skilled individuals who work in complex environments (Allnutt 1987). This model has both advocates (Allnutt 1987; Gaba *et al.* 2003; Helmreich 2000; Howard *et al.* 1992) and detractors (Auerbach *et al.* 2001; Klemola 2000; Norros & Klemola 1999). At issue is the environment of the operating room, which by virtue of the patient, is more complex than an airplane's cockpit (Helmreich 2000). Furthermore, in the aviation model, pilot checklists are used to control all flight and control systems, and are viewed as a

fundamental underpinning of aircraft safety. In contrast, anesthesia safety checklists, although very important, are incomplete as they are primarily oriented toward the anesthesia machine and ventilator, but not cardiovascular monitors, airway equipment, catheters and intravenous lines, infusion pumps, medications, or warming devices (Auerbach *et al.* 2001). Another factor limiting the applicability of the aviation model to anesthesia is that as a general rule, teaching does not occur in the cockpit whereas teaching is prevalent in the operating room (Thomas *et al.* 2004). Regardless of the pros and cons of the aviation model, the important concepts are that the operating room is a complex work environment, made more so by the presence of the patient. Thus, by definition, a veterinary practice, be it small or large, is a complex system. But what other features are the hallmark of complex systems and how do errors occur in them?

In general terms, complex, dynamic environments or systems have the following characteristics (Gaba *et al.* 1994; Woods 1988):

- Incidents unfold in time and are driven by events that occur at indeterminate times. Practically speaking this means that when an incident occurs an individual's ability to problem solve faces a number of challenges, such as pressures of time, overlapping of tasks, requirement for a sustained performance, the changing nature of the problem, and the fact that monitoring can be continuous or semi-continuous, and can change over time.
- Complex systems are made up of highly interconnected parts, and the failure of a single part can have multiple consequences. If we consider the operating room, the loss of electricity would affect a multitude of individuals (surgeon, anesthetist, technicians) and devices (monitoring equipment, cautery, surgical lighting). Our patients are complexity personified. For example, a hypotensive crisis places a patient's heart, kidneys, and brain at risk of failure, which can lead to failure of other organ systems; couple hypotension with hypoxia and the complexity with which we deal during anesthesia becomes quickly apparent.
- When there is high uncertainty in such systems, available data can be ambiguous, incomplete, erroneous, have low signal to noise ratio, or be imprecise with respect to the situation. For example, monitoring devices such as indirect blood pressure monitors, can provide erroneous information, especially during hypo- or hypertensive crises.
- When there is risk, possible outcomes of choices made can have large costs.
- Complex systems can have complex subsystems.

Furthermore, systems possess two general characteristics that predispose to errors: complexity of interactions and tightness of coupling (Gaba *et al.* 1987). Interactions can be of two types. Routine interactions are those that are expected, occur in familiar sequence, and are visible (obvious) even if unplanned. Complex interactions are of unfamiliar sequences, or are unplanned and of unexpected sequences, and are not visible or not immediately comprehensible. Within complex interactions there are three types of complexity (Gaba *et al.* 1987):

1 **Intrinsic complexity:** the physical process is only achieved using a high-technology system that uses precision components acting in a closely coordinated fashion (e.g., space flight and nuclear power).

2 **Proliferation complexity:** the physical process, although simple, requires a large number of simple components (wires, pipes, switches, and valves) interconnected in a very complex fashion (e.g., electrical grids, chemical plants).

3 **Uncertainty complexity:** the physical process is achieved simply but is poorly understood, cause-effect relationships are not clear-cut, have a high degree of unpredictability, and the means of describing and monitoring the process are limited or are of uncertain predictive value (e.g., anesthesia).

Using the airplane pilot as a model of the anesthetist within a complex, dynamic system, M.F. Allnutt describes the anesthetist as "a highly trained professional who uses highly technical equipment, is a member of a team for which the time of work and work conditions are not always ideal, and who uses a high level of cognitive skills in a complex domain about which much is known, but about which much remains to be discovered" (Allnutt 1987). Within this model, human error is synonymous with pilot error. But the pilot may be taking the blame for the individual or individuals who created the error-generating conditions: the manager, trainer, aircraft designer, or ground controller (Allnutt 1987). In other words, it is the individual at the sharp end of a process who takes the blame for mistakes and errors made hours, days, or months earlier by other persons at the blunt managerial end; the individual at the sharp end is only the final common pathway for an error, thrust there by a flawed system (see Case 5.1) (Allnutt 1987). Applying the pilot analogy to an anesthetist, human error in anesthesia may be attributable to the anesthetist, but it may be equally attributable to the anesthetist's trainer, the person who failed to pass on a message to the anesthetist concerning patient- or system-related issues, or the person who designed, bought, or authorized the purchase of an inadequate piece of equipment (Allnutt 1987).

Anesthesia involves the use of drugs that have complications, both known and idiosyncratic (Keats 1979). In an attempt to overcome the **uncertainty complexity** inherent in anesthesia, extensive monitoring may be used, but this in turn generates substantial **proliferation complexity**. A large number of monitors, which may or may not be specific for or sufficiently sensitive to detect a problem early, may overwhelm the anesthetist with data not all of which provide useful information. Indeed, the environment in which anesthetists work may be data-rich but information-poor (Beck & Lin 2003). In fact, when many monitors and drug delivery devices are in use simultaneously there is a high probability that a single component will fail, and the complexity of the interaction between equipment, anesthetist, and patient may be hidden until unmasked by a failure (Gaba *et al.* 1987).

Coupling refers to the degree of interaction or linkage between components of a system (Gaba *et al.* 1987; Webster 2005). Components are loosely coupled when there is a great deal of slack or buffer between them such that a change in one component slowly or minimally affects another component. A loosely coupled system is more forgiving of error and allows greater opportunity for an error to be corrected in time to avoid serious consequences (Webster 2005). In contrast, components that are tightly coupled have very little slack or buffer, and a change in one component quickly or directly affects another (Gaba *et al.* 1987). Thus, tightly coupled systems result in more adverse incidents because minor mistakes or slips can become amplified in their effects before a mistake can be corrected (Webster 2005). An anesthetized patient is a decidedly more tightly coupled system than an awake individual, as many normally self-regulating physiological subsystems have been suspended, altered, or taken over by the technology of the anaesthetic (Webster 2005). For example, at sub-anesthetic levels the ventilatory response (in terms of minute ventilation; L min^{-1}) of a patient breathing a gas mixture low in oxygen is significantly depressed and becomes more depressed as anesthetic depth increases (Hirshman *et al.* 1977). Anesthetists know that during anesthesia various physiological components, such as oxygenation and ventilation, become more tightly coupled. Recognizing that anesthesia tightens coupling, anesthetists use techniques to loosen coupling between components so as to create a greater margin of safety for the patient. Continuing with the example of anesthesia and ventilation, the simple technique of pre-oxygenating patients prior to induction of anesthesia builds up a reservoir of oxygen in the patient so that if apnea occurs during induction the patient has a sufficient oxygen reserve to draw upon until spontaneous or mechanical ventilation commences.

What, then, are errors within complex environments? There are a number of definitions, the most common are:

- Errors are performances that deviate from normal or from the ideal (Allnutt 1987).
- Errors are all occasions in which a planned sequence of mental or physical activities fail to achieve their intended outcome (Reason 1990).
- Errors are failure of a planned action to be completed as intended (i.e., error of execution), or the use of a wrong plan to achieve an aim (i.e., error of planning) (Leape 2002). **This is the definition we use throughout this text.**

These definitions, although broad in scope, do not explain how errors occur. One way of getting to "why" and "how" is to divide errors into two broad categories:

1 **Active errors**, **failures**, or **conditions**—those errors made by operators directly involved in the provision of care (e.g., administering the wrong drug to a patient) and that create weaknesses or absences in or among protective mechanisms in a system (Garnerin *et al.* 2002; Reason 2004; Reason 2005). They are those errors that usually immediately precede an incident.

2 **Latent failures** or **conditions** (also known as root causes, resident pathogens, or James Reason's "bad stuff" (Reason 2004))—those errors waiting to happen because they exist in the environment or system well before the occurrence of an incident.

Three taxonomic categories have been used to describe active errors: **contextual**, **modal**, and **psychological** (Reason 2005; Runciman *et al.* 1993).

A **contextual model** describes errors in terms of particular actions performed in a particular environment (Runciman *et al.* 1993). Using this model, errors in anesthesia would be analyzed based on whether an error occurred during induction, intubation, maintenance, or recovery. This model cannot be applied across different types of environments because it is specific to the anesthetist's domain, so it cannot be a general predictive account of errors; it is only suitable for particular tasks in a particular work environment (Runciman *et al.* 1993).

The **modal model** is a more generalized approach to errors, one that expects errors of omission, substitution, insertion, and repetition to occur in complex systems (Runciman *et al.* 1993). This taxonomy allows one to gain an idea of how frequently a particular type of error, such as substitution, occurs across a variety of systems, but it will not explain how that mode of error manifests itself (Runciman *et al.* 1993).

The **psychological model** tries to describe where in an individual's cognitive processes the error occurred and why it occurred (Runciman *et al.* 1993). This approach is broadly applicable across all circumstances if we recognize, as we should, that errors are actions that have failed, and actions are the results of decisions made (cognitive processes). Thus it follows that we need to look at cognitive processes as the underlying sources of errors (Leape 1994; Stiegler *et al.* 2012; Wheeler & Wheeler 2005). However, as this discussion has shown, errors occur not just as a result of human cognition and action, but as a result of multiple factors existing outside of the individual, including technical, environmental, and organizational. These factors are more fully discussed in the next chapter.

Conclusion

Errors occur not just as a result of human cognition and action, but also as a result of multiple factors existing outside of the individual, including technical, environmental, and organizational factors. The next chapter reviews these factors in greater depth so as to describe more fully how and why errors occur.

References

Allnutt, M.F. (1987) Human factors in accidents. *British Journal of Anaesthesia* **59**(7): 856–864.

Auerbach, A.D., Muff, H.J., & Islam, S.D. (2001) Pre-anesthesia checklists to improve patient safety. In: *Making Health Care Safer: A Critical Analysis of Patient Safety Practices* (eds K.G. Shojania, B.W. Duncan, K.M. McDonald & R.M. Wachter). Rockville, MD: Agency for Health Care Research and Quality, pp. 259–263.

Beck, M.B. & Lin, Z. (2003) Transforming data into information. *Water Science and Technology* **47**(2): 43–51.

Chang, A., *et al.* (2005) The JCAHO patient safety event taxonomy: A standardized terminology and classification schema for near misses and adverse events. *International Journal for Quality in Health Care* **17**(2): 95–105.

Gaba, D.M., *et al.* (1987) Anesthetic mishaps: Breaking the chain of accident evolution. *Anesthesiology* **66**: 670–676.

Gaba, D.M., Fish, K.J., & Howard, S.K. (1994) *Crisis Management in Anesthesiology*. Philadelphia: Churchill Livingstone.

Gaba, D.M., *et al.* (2003) Differences in safety climate between hospital personnel and naval aviators. *Human Factors* **45**(2): 173–185.

Garnerin, P., *et al.* (2002) Root-cause analysis of an airway filter occlusion: A way to improve the reliability of the respiratory circuit. *British Journal of Anaesthesia* **89**(4): 633–635.

Helmreich, R.L. (2000) On error management: Lessons from aviation. *British Medical Journal* **320**(7237): 781–785.

Hirshman, C.A., *et al.* (1977) Depression of hypoxic ventilatory response by halothane, enflurane and isoflurane in dogs. *British Journal of Anaesthesia* **49**(10): 957–963.

Howard, S.K., *et al.* (1992) Anesthesia crisis resource management training: Teaching anesthesiologists to handle critical incidents. *Aviation Space and Environmental Medicine* **63**(9): 763–770.

Keats, A.S. (1979) What do we know about anesthetic mortality? *Anesthesiology* **50**: 387–392.

Klemola, U.M. (2000) The psychology of human error revisited. *Eur J Anaesthesiology* **17**(6): 401–401.

Kohn, L.T., Corrigan, J.M., & Donaldson, M.S. (eds) (2000) *To Err is Human: Building a Safer Health System*. Washington, DC: National Academy Press.

Leape, L.L. (1994) Error in medicine. *Journal of the American Medical Association* **272**(23): 1851–1857.

Leape, L.L. (2002) Reporting of adverse events. *New England Journal of Medicine* **347**(20): 1633–1638.

Norros, L. & Klemola, U. (1999) Methodological considerations in analysing anaesthetists' habits of action in clinical situations. *Ergonomics* **42**(11): 1521–1530.

Reason, J.T. (1990) *Human Error*. Cambridge: Cambridge University Press.

Reason, J.T. (2004) Beyond the organisational accident: The need for "error wisdom" on the frontline. *Quality and Safety in Health Care* **13**(Suppl. 2): ii28–ii33.

Reason, J.T. (2005) Safety in the operating theatre – part 2: Human error and organisational failure. *Quality and Safety in Health Care* **14**(1): 56–60.

Runciman, W.B., *et al.* (1993) Errors, incidents and accidents in anaesthetic practice. *Anaesthesia and Intensive Care* **21**(5): 506–519.

Runciman, W., *et al.* (2009) Towards an international classification for patient safety: Key concepts and terms. *International Journal for Quality in Health Care* **21**(1): 18–26.

Sherman, H., *et al.* (2009) Towards an international classification for patient safety: The conceptual framework. *International Journal for Quality in Health Care* **21**(1): 2–8.

Stiegler, M.P., *et al.* (2012) Cognitive errors detected in anesthesiology: A literature review and pilot study. *British Journal of Anaesthesia* **108**(2): 229–235.

Thomas, E.J., *et al.* (2004) Translating teamwork behaviours from aviation to healthcare: Development of behavioural markers for neonatal resuscitation. *Quality and Safety in Health Care* **13**(Suppl. 1): i57–i64.

Thomson, R., *et al.* (2009) Towards an international classification for patient safety: A delphi survey. *International Journal for Quality in Health Care* **21**(1): 9–17.

Webster, C.S. (2005) The nuclear power industry as an alternative analogy for safety in anaesthesia and a novel approach for the conceptualisation of safety goals. *Anaesthesia* **60**(11): 1115–1122.

Wheeler, S.J. & Wheeler, D.W. (2005) Medication errors in anaesthesia and critical care. *Anaesthesia* **60**(3): 257–273.

WHO (2009) *Conceptual Framework for the International Classification for Patient Safety - Final Technical Report January 2009*. World Health Organization.

Woods, D.D. (1988) Coping with complexity: the psychology of human behavior in complex systems. In: *Tasks, Errors and Mental Models* (eds L.P. Goodstein, H.B. Andersen, & S.E. Olsen). London: Taylor & Francis, pp. 128–148.

CHAPTER 2

Errors: Organizations, Individuals, and Unsafe Acts

Errors at the sharp end are symptomatic of both human fallibility and underlying organizational failings. Fallibility is here to stay. Organizational and local problems, in contrast, are both diagnosable and manageable.

James Reason (2005)

Rather than being the instigators of an accident, operators tend to be the inheritors of system defect…their part is usually that of adding the final garnish to a lethal brew whose ingredients have already been long in the cooking.

James Reason (1990b)

While observing the aftermath of an incident that caused the death of a patient, a colleague commented, "I can't even imagine this error happening." Unfortunately the unimaginable often occurs when local conditions necessary for error generation exist within the work environment and are triggered—activated—by actions taken at the human-system interface (Reason 1990b). In reality, everything we humans devise, use, or do is prone to error and failure (Haerkens *et al.* 2015). So where do we begin in order to gain an understanding of how errors occur so that we can prevent them? To answer this question we have drawn heavily on the model developed by James Reason (Reason 1990a, 1990b) and subsequently adapted by others specifically to address errors and adverse incidents in medicine (Diller *et al.* 2014; Karsh *et al.* 2006; Leape 1994; Vincent *et al.* 1998, 2014). These models are based on systems and human factors analysis approaches, which focus on multiple error-generating factors found at the organizational, supervisory, environmental, personnel, and individual levels.

We have drawn on these models and modified them with the goal of characterizing the environment within which veterinary anesthetists work, an environment that includes technical, organizational, and human factors domains and the multiplicity of factors in those domains involved in error generation (Figure 2.1). In Figure 2.1 the domains are bounded by broken lines so as to reflect the real world in which anesthetists work;

a world in which elements within and outside the work environment can influence our practice of anesthesia and yet are often beyond our control. The arrows between the various elements are bi-directional reflecting the fact that these interactions are two-way, one influencing the other and vice versa. This environmental model serves as the outline for this chapter.

Error causation: technical factors

Errors do occur as a result of technical or equipment failures, but they are infrequent (Reason 2005). This is not to belittle or ignore these types of failures, especially when they harm either a patient or a healthcare provider. An issue with technical or equipment failures is how to quickly identify and correct these types of errors when they occur so that they do not cause further patient harm. Chapter 4 presents a few cases involving equipment failures, how they were detected, and strategies that were used to quickly identify them.

Error causation: organizational and supervision factors

Before discussing this topic in depth we need to ask, is a discussion of organizations relevant to veterinary medicine? More specifically, are private veterinary practices

Errors in Veterinary Anesthesia, First Edition. John W. Ludders and Matthew McMillan.
© 2017 John Wiley & Sons, Inc. Published 2017 by John Wiley & Sons, Inc.

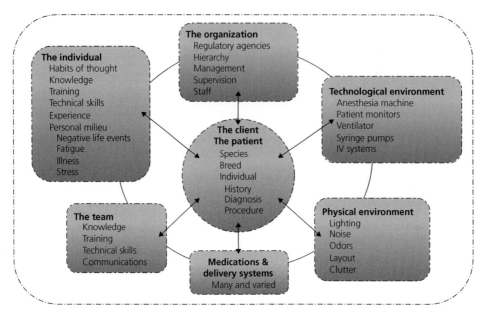

Figure 2.1 This graphic shows the environment within which a veterinary anesthetist functions when managing an anesthetized patient. The outermost and all inner borders are broken lines that reflect the real world in which we work, a world in which elements within and outside our work environment, often beyond our control, can influence our practice of anesthesia. The arrows between the various elements are bi-directional reflecting the fact that these interactions are two-way, one influencing the other and vice versa. It contains Reason's factors involved in making unsafe acts, including the organization, the individual, the team, the physical and technological environments, and medications and their delivery systems.

organizations? Probably we would agree that multi-veterinarian practices, such as referral practices/hospitals and university teaching hospitals, are organizations, but what about single- or two-veterinarian practices? An organization is defined as:

> …a body of people structured and managed to meet a specific goal; as such it has a management structure that determines relationships between the different activities and members of the organization, and assigns roles, responsibilities, and authority to carry out different tasks. *Organizations are open systems that affect and are affected by their environment* (our emphasis).
>
> *Modified from: http://www.businessdictionary.com/ definition/organization.html (accessed November 8, 2015)*

We contend that these organizational elements exist in all veterinary practices, be they large or small in size. That said, it is important to note that each veterinary practice, be it a single- or multi-person practice, has its own unique ways of accomplishing the day-to-day tasks inherent in its operation. These routine tasks, often referred to as "standard operating procedures," may be routine for one practice but not for another. These aspects of the practice directly or indirectly affect all

aspects of patient management, including anesthesia. A procedure or process deeply embedded in one practice may not even exist in another practice. What may raise a question in the mind of a visitor to a practice may not even seem worthy of consideration by those working within the practice because "it's just the way we do things here"; it is part and parcel of the organization's culture.

So what role does the organization play? It is true that people make errors or at the very least are the final common pathway by which errors occur. But people do not go to work intending to make errors or cause harm. Error generation is often due to organization-related factors inherent in the organization and that influence the behavior and action of those within it (Battles & Shea 2001; Garnerin *et al.* 2002; Klemola 2000; Kruskal *et al.* 2008; Reason 2004; Wald & Shojania 2001). A number of terms have been used to describe these factors, including **latent conditions** or **latent failures** (also known as **root causes** or **"resident pathogens"**). These conditions exist as a result of defensive gaps, weaknesses, or absences unwittingly created in a system due to earlier decisions made by the designers, builders, regulators, managers, and supervisors of the organization or system. Examples of latent conditions include vials of similar shape, size, and color containing entirely different drugs; or similar labels for two different drugs (for an example see Case 5.1) (Garnerin *et al.* 2002; Reason 2004).

Latent conditions possess two important properties: their effects are usually longer lasting than those created by active failures (the latter are failures that occur due to actions taken by individuals at the human-system interface); and they exist within the system prior to an adverse event. These two properties mean that latent conditions can be detected and repaired before they cause harm (Reason 2004) As such, latent conditions are the primary targets of any safety management system (Reason 2004).

Management, too, has a role in error generation. For example, those at the frontlines of healthcare may be the recipients of a variety of latent failures attributable to supervision. In these situations there may be failure of leadership exemplified by inadequate training, or lack of professional guidance or oversight, all of which encourage non-standard approaches to patient care (Diller *et al.* 2014). There may be a lack of operational planning, a failure to correct known problems, or inadequate or missing supervisory ethics such as turning a blind eye to violations of standard operating procedures. Resource management such as the allocation and maintenance of organizational resources, including human resources, monetary budgets, and equipment design, can create latent conditions that set the stage for error generation.

Corporate decisions about allocation of such resources usually focus on two objectives: (1) quality of the work, and (2) on-time and cost-effective operations. In many situations quality is sacrificed for cost control or efficiency thus setting the stage for adverse incidents (Diller *et al.* 2014). This concept is perhaps best outlined by Hollnagel's Efficiency-Thoroughness Trade-Off (ETTO) principle (Hollnagel 2009). In general, this principle refers to the idea that during their daily activities individuals and organizations must make "trade-offs" between the resources (time, effort, personnel, etc.) they expend on preparing, planning, and monitoring an activity (their thoroughness) and the resources (again time, effort, personnel, etc.) they expend on performing the activity (their efficiency). Safety conscious individuals and organizations favor thoroughness over efficiency, while those favoring productivity favor efficiency over thoroughness. The ETTO principle makes the assumption that it is impossible to maximize both thoroughness and efficiency at the same time and recognizes that an activity will not succeed without some degree of both. Hollnagel gives a number of reasons commonly used to justify making ETTO decisions, including "it is normally OK, there is no need to check because it will be checked later," or "we always do it this way," or "this way is much quicker." Our experiences suggest that these formal and informal organizational processes, such as operational tempo, time pressures, schedules, and balancing thoroughness against efficiency, also occur in veterinary anesthesia and give a sense of the influence organizational climate can have on the individual and culture of patient safety.

Senior management should ensure that the organization's culture and climate focuses on patient safety. This can be accomplished through operational processes, including formal processes, procedures, and oversight within the organization. All of this implies that an organization with a culture attuned to error prevention and patient safety is willing and able to learn from errors. This state of organizational being has been variously described as that of the learning organization, or the high reliability organization (HRO) (Sutcliffe 2011). These organizations are skilled at creating, acquiring, and transferring knowledge and modifying their behavior to reflect new knowledge and insights gained from error reporting and analysis (Palazzolo & Stoutenburgh 1997; Sutcliffe 2011; Vogus & Hilligoss 2015). HROs possess the following essential components (Palazzolo & Stoutenburgh 1997; Sutcliffe 2011):

- **Systems thinking**—individuals within the organization recognize that dynamic complexity in complex systems means that problems are a meshwork of interrelated actions.
- **Personal mastery**—there is a continuous process and state of mind that enables individuals within the learning organization to master a discipline.
- **Mental models**—individuals recognize that they have biased images of reality and that they can challenge those views and develop different views or models of reality.
- **Building shared visions**—a shared view of the organization's vision is developed so that it fosters genuine commitment to the vision, not just compliance.

- **Team learning**—teams are the fundamental learning unit of the organization for it is in teams that views of reality are shared and assumptions are challenged and tested.

A learning organization is also distinguished by how it acts (**heedful interrelating**) and what it does (**heedful attending**), both of which lead to **mindful performance** (Weick 2002). According to Weick, heedful attending is embodied in five processes (Weick 2002):

1 A preoccupation with failure such that the people assume each day will be a bad day and act accordingly.
2 A reluctance to simplify interpretations because they know that hubris is their enemy, and optimism is the height of arrogance.
3 A sensitivity to operations so as to maintain situational awareness.
4 Commitment to resilience and the ability to cope with unanticipated dangers after they have occurred, and do so by paying close attention to their ability to investigate, learn, and act without prior knowledge of what they will be called upon to act on.
5 A willingness to organize around expertise thus letting those with the expertise make decisions.

Somewhat taking liberties here, the flip side of the learning organization might be what Reason calls the **vulnerable system** (Reason *et al.* 2001). A vulnerable system or organization is one that displays the "**vulnerable system syndrome**" (VSS) and its cluster of pathologies that render it more liable to experience errors and adverse incidents. Reason describes the syndrome as possessing three interacting and self-perpetuating characteristics: (1) blaming errors on front-line individuals; (2) denying the existence of systemic error-provoking weaknesses; and (3) the blinkered pursuit of productive and financial indicators (Reason *et al.* 2001). However, Reason also states:

> Even the most resistant organizations can suffer a bad accident. By the same token, even the most vulnerable systems can evade disaster, at least for a time. Chance does not take sides. It afflicts the deserving and preserves the unworthy.
>
> *Reason (2000).*

It is unwise to define success based on a chance occurrence. In anesthesia, success in safety means that an outcome is achieved by minimizing the risk of harm without relying on the quick wits of the anesthetist,

a robust patient, and a pinch of good fortune; that is, it should not be defined merely as having an alive and conscious patient at the end of anesthesia.

This brings us to **resilience** in healthcare systems. Resilience is the intrinsic ability of a system to adjust its functioning in response to changes in circumstances so that it can continue to function successfully, even after an adverse incident, or in the presence of continuous stress or latent conditions. It revolves around clinicians' abilities to make appropriate judgments regarding when and how to follow control measures and how the existing system supports this decision-making process. Resilience is the manner in which a system is able to respond to unexpected events and meet new demands while buffering challenges to safety. Rather than suppressing human variability by adding more and more control measures, resilience embraces human variability and the ability to make moment-to-moment adaptations and adjustments in the face of changing events in an uncertain and dynamic world (Reason 2000). There are many hallmarks of a resilient organization, including its culture and subcultures, which shape the organization's ability to meaningfully confront errors wherever and whenever they occur and to learn from them (see "Developing a safety culture" in Chapter 8). Resilience is an important aspect of error prevention within an organization.

Leape states that error prevention efforts must focus on system-associated errors that occur as a result of design, and that design implementation must be considered a part of error prevention (Leape 2002). This approach requires methods of error reduction at each stage of system development, including design, construction, maintenance, allocation of resources, and training and development of operational procedures. The design process must take into consideration the reality that errors will occur and must include plans for recovering from errors. Designs should automatically correct errors when they occur, but when that is not possible, the design should detect errors before they cause harm. This means the system should build in both **buffers** (design features that automatically correct for human or mechanical errors) and **redundancy** (duplication of critical mechanisms and instruments so that failure of a component does not result in loss of function). Tasks should be designed to minimize errors including simplifying and standardizing tasks so as to minimize the load on the weakest aspects of cognition, which are short-term memory, planning, and problem-solving.

Prevention is the process of removing factors (root causes) that contribute to unsafe situations, but it is not the only means for reducing errors (Garnerin *et al.* 2002, 2006; Leape 1994). Another process, that of **absorption**, is intended to eliminate root causes (Reason's "bad stuff"), including cultural causes, such as organizational roadblocks, which hinder early identification and correction of active failures (Garnerin *et al.* 2002, 2006). Absorption involves incorporating buffers into a system so that errors are identified and absorbed or intercepted before they cause patient harm (Garnerin *et al.* 2006; Leape 1994). Using both prevention and absorption enhances the elimination of errors more so than if only one approach is used (Garnerin *et al.* 2002). An example of prevention is a policy that makes it widely known within an organization that there is the potential for a particular type of error to occur. An example of absorption is the adoption of specific techniques or procedures within the organization to specifically prevent the occurrence of the error. A real life example serves to make this point.

In the Equine/Farm Animal Hospital of the Cornell University Hospital for Animals, any large animal patient undergoing anesthesia for any reason is aseptically catheterized intravenously with a 14-gauge, 5.25-inch catheter. These catheters are typically inserted into a patient's jugular vein and secured in place by suturing the catheter hub to the skin; a catheter may remain in a patient for up to 24 to 36 hours depending on postoperative care. The catheter that is the focus of this example is actually designed for use in human patients, not veterinary patients.

In the mid-1990s when these catheters first started to be used in the hospital, it was discovered that partial separation of the catheter shaft from the hub occurred occasionally when removing a catheter from a patient. Unfortunately, in one patient a complete separation occurred and the catheter traveled down the jugular vein and lodged in the patient's lung. The manufacturer was contacted regarding this problem and to the company's credit, company representatives visited the hospital to gain a better understanding of how the catheters were used and the nature of the problem. The manufacturer made some changes in catheter design and assembly and as a result this problem disappeared for a number of years.

The problem unexpectedly reappeared a few years later when, during anesthesia of a horse, the anesthetist noticed that the IV fluids being administered to the patient were leaking from the catheter under the skin and creating a very large fluid-filled subcutaneous mass. The fluids were stopped and another catheter was inserted into the opposite jugular vein so that fluid administration could continue. The defective catheter was removed, inspected, and found to have a hole and tear at the catheter-hub interface (Figure 2.2). A test determined that a needle inserted through the injection cap into the catheter was not long enough to cause the hole and tear, thus the problem was attributed to a flaw in the catheter itself. To prevent harm to other large

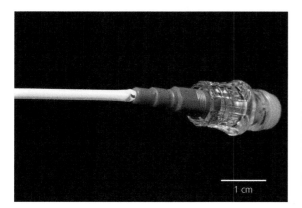 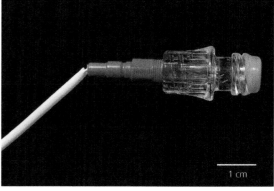

Figure 2.2 Two views of a 14-gauge catheter typically used for intravenous catheterization of horses and cattle. The hole and tear in this catheter was noticed after it was removed from a horse's jugular vein. Had there been more skin-associated drag on the catheter it may well have torn off the hub and traveled down the jugular vein to lodge in the horse's lungs.

animal patients, this problem was dealt with using a two-pronged approach: first, the problem with the catheter was made widely known throughout the Equine/Farm Animal Hospital, specifically at a regularly scheduled monthly meeting that involved all faculty, house officers, and technicians. A technique was also presented to show how to block a catheter from floating down the jugular vein should it tear free from the hub during its removal from a patient. This is an example of the processes of prevention and absorption that when used together increase the likelihood of eliminating hazards within the work environment.

Error causation: environmental factors

Environmental factors include the physical environment with its lighting, noise, smells, clutter, and room layout. It also includes the technological environment with its equipment and control design, display, or interface characteristics.

Error causation: personnel factors

Personnel factors involve communication and information flow, such as miscommunication between individuals or when information is incomplete or unavailable. Other personnel factors include coordination failures that occur when individuals work independently rather than as team members; planning failures that occur when providers fail to anticipate a patient's needs or create inappropriate treatment plans; and issues of fitness for duty, which can include many possibilities, such as sickness, fatigue, and self-medication with licit or illicit drugs that impair function.

Error causation: human factors

Both Reason and Diller use the term "unsafe acts" to describe the actions of those at the human-system interface that cause errors. As previously mentioned, Reason's unsafe acts are due to the basic error types of slips, lapses, and mistakes (Figure 2.3) (Reason 1990a). Diller, drawing on Reason's framework and applying it to healthcare, states that unsafe acts, or active failures, are those actions taken by individuals that cause errors and violations (Diller *et al*. 2014) (Figure 2.4 and Table 2.1). In Diller's approach, errors can be categorized as:

- **Decision errors**—occur when information, knowledge, or experience is lacking.
- **Skill-based errors**—occur when a care provider makes a mistake while engaged in a very familiar task (see Case 5.1). This type of error is particularly susceptible to attention or memory failures, especially when a care giver is interrupted or distracted.

Figure 2.3 This graphic relates unsafe acts to unintended and intended actions and the basic error types and cognitive failures that underlie them. Of special note is that violations are not errors, they are intentional actions that may or may not cause harm. From: James Reason (1990) *Human Error*. Cambridge, UK: Cambridge University Press, p. 207. With permission of the publisher.

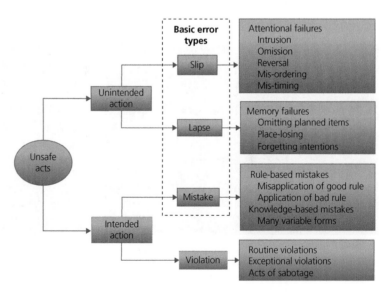

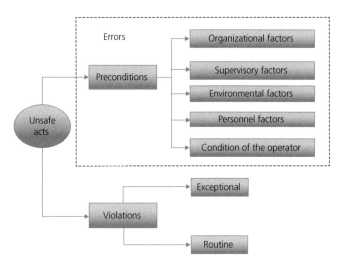

Figure 2.4 This graphic outlines how unsafe acts can lead to errors when any number of preconditions exist within the environment. The preconditions consist of human factors domains as described by Diller *et al*. From: Thomas Diller *et al*. (2014) The Human Factors Analysis Classification System (HFACS) applied to health care. *American Journal of Medical Quality* **29**(3): 181–90. With permission of the publisher.

- **Perceptual errors**—occur when input to one of the five senses is degraded or incomplete, such as poor hearing or eyesight.
- **Violations**—intentional departure from accepted practices, so by definition they are not errors. Violations include **routine violations**, those that are habitual by nature and often enabled by management that tolerates "bending the rules"; and **exceptional violations**, or willful behaviors outside the norms and regulations that are condoned by management, not engaged in by others, and not part of the individual's usual behavior.

Actions taken, regardless of whether intended or unintended, are preceded by cognitive processes, so we must understand the role of cognitive processes in error causation if we want to prevent errors or minimize their effects. Reason (1990a) has developed a cognitive model to explain in general terms how errors occur, and Drs Lucian Leape (1994) and Thomas Diller (Diller *et al*. 2014) have adapted that model to the field of medicine. According to this model, which is based on human cognition, the human mind functions in two modes (Leape 1994; Stanovich 2011; Stiegler *et al*. 2012; Wheeler & Wheeler 2005):

1 **Schematic control mode** (also called **intuitive** or **Type I cognitive processing**)—an automatic, fast-response mode of cognition in which the mind has unconscious mental models composed of old knowledge—schemata—that are activated by very little conscious thought, or activated by sensory inputs that the mind tends to interpret in accordance with the general character of earlier experiences. In this mode thinking (mental functioning) is automatic, rapid, and effortless (Leape 1994). We use intuitive mode for ease of use and understanding.

2 **Attentional control mode** (also called **analytical** or **Type II cognitive processing**)—a controlled, conscious, analytical mode of cognition requiring effort that is difficult to sustain, and uses stored knowledge; it is called into play when a new situation is encountered or the intuitive mode has failed. In this mode of thinking deliberate effort has to be made to determine what information to pay attention to and what to ignore. We use analytical mode for ease of use and understanding.

The intuitive mode is characterized by the use of heuristics, a process of learning, discovery, or problem-solving by trial-and-error methods. It is also a process by which we use cognitive short-cuts—rules of thumb—to reduce the cognitive cost of decision-making (Croskerry *et al*. 2013a; Reason 2008; Stiegler & Tung 2014). If we think of problem-solving, such as making a diagnosis, as being linked by some cognitive pathway to stored knowledge, then heuristics lies along that pathway and is just another way of applying stored knowledge to novel problems; it is neither a faulty (error-prone) nor faultless (error-free) process (McLaughlin *et al*. 2014). In fact, experienced decision makers use heuristics in ways that increase their decision-making efficiency (Kovacs & Croskerry 1999). Heuristics save time and effort in making daily decisions. Indeed, while performing daily activities we spend about 95% of our

Table 2.1 Diller *et al.*'s classification system of factors involved in error generation is based on the Human Factors Analysis Classification System and is intended for application to healthcare. It includes elements of Reason's Generic Errors Model.

Organizational influences

Resource management—allocation failures of organizational resources

Organizational climate—factors that adversely influence worker performance

Organizational processes—failure of formal processes, procedures and oversight

Supervision

Inadequate leadership

Inappropriate planned operations

Failure to correct known problems

Supervisory violations (supervisory ethics)

Preconditions for unsafe acts

Environment factors

   Physical environment

   Technological environment

Personnel factors—provider behavior contributing to an adverse incident

   Communication and information flow

   Coordination failures

   Planning failure

   Fitness for duty—fatigue, illness, self-medication that reduces capability

Condition of the operator

   Adverse mental state

   Adverse physiological state

   Chronic performance limitations

     Lack of knowledge

     Inadequate training

     Lack of experience

     Lack of technical knowledge

Unsafe acts

Errors

   Skill-based—mistake is made while engaged in a very familiar task

   Decision error—information, knowledge, or experience is lacking

   Perceptual error—occurs when one of the five senses is degraded or incomplete

Violations—intentional departures from accepted practice

   Routine—often enabled by management

   Exceptional—behavior outside the norm and not condoned by management

---

From: Thomas Diller *et al.* (2014) The Human Factors Analysis Classification System (HFACS) applied to health care. *American Journal of Medical Quality* **29**(3): 181–90. With permission of the publisher.

time in the intuitive mode using heuristics (Croskerry *et al.* 2013a). This is an acceptable approach when time and circumstances permit, but potentially detrimental in an emergent situation (Croskerry *et al.* 2013a). Cognitive scientists recognize that the human mind prefers to function as a context-specific pattern recognizer rather than use the analytical mode and calculate, analyze, or optimize (Reason 1990a). In fact, we humans prefer pattern matching over calculation to such a degree that we are strongly biased to search for a pre-packaged solution before resorting to a more strenuous knowledge-based level of performance (Leape 1994). Thus we have a prevailing disposition to use heuristics. While it works well most of the time, heuristics can lead to errors in decision-making, including clinical decision-making, due to the influence of biases (Croskerry *et al.* 2013a; Hall 2002).

The analytical mode is used for conscious problem-solving that is required when a problem is confronted that has not been encountered before or as a result of failures of the intuitive mode. It requires more cognitive effort and draws upon stored knowledge and past experience to aid decision-making (Leape 1994).

Within this cognitive model three levels of human performance have been identified and used in error analysis (Leape 1994; Reason 1990a):

1 **Skill-based (SB) level performance** is governed by stored patterns of preprogrammed instructions—schemata—that are largely unconscious, characterized as highly routinized, and occur in familiar circumstances. Skill-based performance relates to technical performance and proper execution of tasks (Kruskal *et al.* 2008).

2 **Rule-based (RB) level performance** consists of actions or solutions governed by stored rules of the type *if…then*. Rule-based performance requires conscious thought; it relates to supervision, training and qualifications, communication, and interpretation (Kruskal *et al.* 2008).

3 **Knowledge-based (KB) level performance** occurs when synthetic thought is used for novel situations. This level of performance requires conscious analytical processing and stored knowledge, and it requires effort.

Conceiving of and executing an action sequence involves the cognitive processes of **planning, storage** (memory), and **execution**. Errors can occur within any of these three stages, and the types of errors are characterized as **slips**, **lapses**, or **mistakes**—Reason's basic error types. Slips are actions that occur not as planned even though the intended action may have been correct, that is, the actual execution of the action was wrong. Slips are usually observable (usually overt). As an aside, slips have been described as failures of low-level mental processing (Allnutt 1987). This terminology—"low-level mental processing"—is not a reflection of intelligence nor is it meant to be derogatory, but recognizes that an individual who makes a slip is distracted by any number of possible causes, and his or her full attention is not on the task at hand. Absent-minded slips increase the likelihood of making errors of omission, that is, failing to take a required action (Reason 1990a).

Lapses involve failures of memory that occur when an individual's attention is distracted or preoccupied. They are usually apparent only to the person who experiences them (Reason 1990a). Both slips and lapses occur at the skill-based level (Reason 1990a).

Mistakes, on the other hand, occur when a plan is inadequate to achieve its desired goal even though the actions may run according to plan; mistakes occur at the planning stage of both rule-based and knowledge-based levels of performance (Helmreich 2000; Reason 1990b, 2005). Rule-based errors (mistakes) occur when a good rule is misapplied because an individual fails to interpret the situation correctly, or a bad rule that exists in memory is applied to the situation (Reason 2005).

Knowledge-based errors (mistakes) are complex in nature because it is difficult to identify what an individual was actually thinking, what the cognitive processes were, prior to and at the time of an error. The usual scenario is that a novel situation is encountered for which the individual does not possess prepro-grammed solutions (no schemata) and an error arises for lack of knowledge, or because the problem is misinterpreted. Mistakes have been described as failures of higher level cognition, that is, failure of the analytical mode of cognition (Allnutt 1987). Mistakes occur as a result of the same physiological, psychological (including stress), and environmental factors that produce slips (see Figure 2.3).

Leape has somewhat modified Reason's model by focusing only on slips and mistakes and considers lapses to be slips (Box 2.1). According to Leape (1994), slips are unintended acts. Usually the operator has the requisite skills, but there is a lack of a timely attentional check, so slips are failures of self-monitoring. This phrase—"failures of self-monitoring"—implies that the individual is solely responsible for the slip, but often slips occur as a result of factors that distract or divert the individual's attention from the task at hand. Leape has identified a number of attention-diverting factors, or distractions, most of which are familiar to everyone in veterinary medicine, not just in veterinary anesthesia (Leape 1994):

- **Physiological**—fatigue, sleep loss, alcohol or drug abuse, illness.

Box 2.1 The types of slips described by Leape (1994) and modified with examples from veterinary anesthesia.

- **Capture slips**—for example, when providing a manual sigh to an anesthetized patient the usual sequence of actions is to partially or completely close the pop-off valve (adjustable pressure limiting valve—APL) on the circle breathing circuit of the anesthesia machine, squeeze the reservoir bag until the airway pressure reaches some predetermined limit, release the reservoir bag, fully open the pop-off valve, check the patient, and continue with anesthetic management. If the anesthetist is distracted just after sighing the patient there is a high likelihood that he or she will forget to open the pop-off valve, a known problem in veterinary anesthesia (Hofmeister *et al.* 2014). This slip becomes apparent when the anesthetist observes the distended reservoir bag, or high airway pressure develops and causes cardiopulmonary collapse in the patient.

- **Description slips**—in this type of error the correct action is performed on the wrong object. For example, an anesthetist may reach for the oxygen flowmeter control knob on an anesthesia machine with the intent of increasing oxygen flow, but instead grasps the nitrous oxide flow control knob and increases the flow of nitrous oxide.

- **Associative activation slips**—in this type of slip there is a mental association of ideas such as checking one's cell phone when a monitor sounds an alarm.

- **Loss of activation slips**—a well-recognized example is when a person enters a room to do something but cannot remember what it was, i.e., there is a temporary memory loss. Although sometimes jokingly referred to as a "senior moment," this type of slip can occur in any person regardless of age (oh, what a relief!).

- **Psychological** (may be internal or external of the individual)—other activity (busyness), emotional states such as boredom, frustration, fear, anxiety, anger, or depression.
- **Environmental**—noise, heat, visual stimuli, odors, motion, clutter, room layout.

Diller has expanded attention-diverting factors to include personnel factors, which include **coordination failures** and **planning failures**, and communication and information flow (Diller *et al.* 2014). Communications, especially breakdowns in communication, need more discussion because of their role in error causation.

Communication: what it is and how it fails

According to the Institute of Medicine, up to 98,000 patients die and another 15 million are harmed annually in US hospitals due to medical errors (Kohn *et al.* 2000). Root cause analysis has revealed that up to 84% of errors are due to communication failures (Nagpal *et al.* 2012; Welch *et al.* 2013), and that communication failures by human healthcare professionals significantly increase patient morbidity and mortality (Nagpal *et al.* 2012).

Communication is the process by which information is passed from one individual to another, but it can break down in one of three ways (Lingard *et al.* 2004):

1 **Source failure**—information never transmitted such that information is missing or incomplete, e.g., failing to enter a note on a patient's medical record that it has a history of aggression.
2 **Transmission failure**—information misunderstood or transmitted poorly in that a poor method or structure is used for communication, e.g., illegible handwriting.
3 **Receiver failure**—information is forgotten, inaccurately received, or interpreted incorrectly, e.g., information overload overwhelms the receiver's short-term memory and an important detail of patient care is forgotten.

Breakdowns in communication can occur in terms of their **occasion**, **content**, **audience**, or **purpose**. An occasion failure is a problem with the situation or context within which the communication occurs (Box 2.2).

A content failure occurs when the information being communicated is inadequate because it is incomplete, inaccurate, or overly complicated thus leading to information overload or confusion (Box 2.3).

Box 2.2 Example of an occasion failure.

Surgeon [prior to making first incision]: "Have we checked that there is blood in the fridge? I've only just been able to review the images and this may bleed a lot."

Problem: Although sensible to check on the availability of blood this communication has occurred after the patient is anesthetized, is in the OR, and the first incision is about to be made. This communication comes too late to serve as either a prompt or safety redundancy measure. What happens if blood is not available? Either the procedure is aborted, or it continues with the hope that the patient does not bleed significantly. Either way patient safety has been compromised.

Box 2.3 Example of a content failure.

A new employee in an emergency practice is unfamiliar with the practice's standard operating procedures, facilities, and equipment, and is told to attach an oxygen insufflation hose to the endotracheal tube that has been inserted into the trachea of a German shepherd dog. The employee inserts the hose into the ETT rather than attach it to a flow-by device; oxygen flow is set at 5 L min^{-1} and causes a pneumothorax.

Problem: The communication was incomplete as it did not include any further instructions or guidance to the new employee (see Preface).

An audience failure occurs when the make-up of the group involved in the communication is incomplete, that is, a person or people vital to the situation are missing (Box 2.4).

A failure in purpose occurs when the purpose of the communication is not made clear or is not achieved (Box 2.5).

How big is the communication problem in the operating room (OR)?

Communication breakdowns are recognized as a major cause of error and inefficiency in operating rooms (Table 2.2). An observational study identified 421 communication events in 48 human surgical cases, nearly one-third of which were communication failures (Lingard *et al.* 2004). The study concluded that communication failures are "frequent in the OR, occurring in

Box 2.4 Example of an audience failure.

Internist: "We need to perform a bronchoscopy this afternoon."
Anesthetist: "That's fine! We have a couple of slots available, either 1 p.m. or 3 p.m.?
Internist: "OK, I'll see you at 3 p.m. I have a recheck consult at 1 p.m."

Problem: At first glance this seems fine until we consider that the technician/nurse responsible for the scope is not included in this communication. Although the availability of an anesthesiologist has been confirmed, the availability of a room, scope, and technician/nurse required to assist has not. Without being present during this communication either the technician/nurse will fail to be informed in time or a separate communication event will need to occur. Neither is ideal.

Box 2.5 Examples of a failure in purpose.

EXAMPLE 1

Nurse [performing a pre-induction checklist]: "Are antibiotics to be given?"
Anesthetist: "I don't know, it doesn't say on the form."
Nurse: "They often don't for this type of procedure, shall I page the surgeon?"
Anesthetist: "No. Let's move on; I don't want to delay things."

Problem: In this case, the purpose of the communication—to find out whether to administer antibiotics—was not achieved and no action was made to remedy it.

EXAMPLE 2

Anesthetist: "Has owner consent been gained? Being a medical referral it was obviously admitted without surgery in mind."
Surgery resident: "Dr X was going to phone after rounds, so we can crack on."

Problem: In this situation owner consent for surgery has not been confirmed and will only be confirmed after the patient has been anesthetized.

approximately 30% of procedurally relevant exchanges amongst team members and can lead to inefficiency, tension, delay, workaround violations of recognized good practice, waste of resources, patient inconvenience and procedural error" (Lingard *et al.* 2004). Another

observational study of general surgery cases found communication breakdowns or information loss in all of the cases (Christian *et al.* 2006). And in a review of 444 surgical malpractice cases 60 involved communication breakdowns that had a significant role in the adverse outcomes (Greenberg *et al.* 2007). Each case contained between one and six separate communication breakdowns, split evenly between the pre-, intra-, and postoperative periods. The vast majority occurred in communications between two individuals, most commonly between surgeon and anesthetist, and between clinician and trainee (Christian *et al.* 2006; Nagpal *et al.* 2012). It appears that communication failures are a cause of both near misses and adverse incidents, often involving those at the very top of the decision-making tree.

Causes of communication breakdowns and errors have been categorized into task and technology factors, team factors, individual factors, environmental factors, and organizational factors (Nagpal *et al.* 2012). Transferring information using an inadequate form of communication was the primary task and technology factor. For example, information can be transferred on forms that are unsuitable for the task or lack proper structure, that is, there is a lack of protocol or standardization as to how information should be transferred. Another task and technology factor is the information itself, such as laboratory results or imaging reports, being stored in an inappropriate location and unavailable to those requiring the information (e.g., a report is in a clinician's mailbox rather than the patient's file).

Hierarchy also obstructs the flow of information from junior staff members to senior staff members (Greenberg *et al.* 2007). Poor leadership and ambiguity about roles and responsibilities during a task are teamwork factors that can affect communication (Greenberg *et al.* 2007). Factors attributable to individuals include: forgetting information that has been properly transmitted (memory lapses); different levels of staff experience and competency; and junior and assistant staff not feeling empowered to play an active role in patient care. Environmental factors include distractions and high workload, while organizational factors include staffing inadequacies (inadequate numbers, lack of training, poorly defined roles, or rapid turnover), or too many steps and tasks in the system (too many forms and administrative hoops to jump through).

Table 2.2 A set of themes and types of communication failures that occur at various stages of the perioperative period and are based on an analysis of communication failures in the operating room.

- **Pre-op assessment**
  - ○ Source failures
    - Information in different locations
    - Consent/notes/reports missing
    - Documentation inadequate
  - ○ Transmission failures
    - Lack of communication between anesthesia and surgical teams
    - Information not relayed from pre-assessment to OR
  - ○ Receiver failures
    - Specialist's opinion not checked
- **Pre-procedural**
  - ○ Source failures
    - Schedule changed multiple times
    - Incorrect/incomplete name on schedule
  - ○ Transmission failures
    - Lack of briefing
    - No collaboration between teams
  - Lack of communication between wards and OR
  - ○ Receiver failures
    - Equipment/ICU bed availability not checked
    - Checklists not followed

- **Post-operative**
  - ○ Source failures
    - Hand-off incomplete
    - Illegible written instructions
    - Too much information
  - ○ Transmission failures
    - Lack of debriefing
    - Notes not transferred
  - ○ Receiver failures
    - Multi-tasking or distractions occurring during hand-offs, partial receiving of information
- **Daily ward care**
  - ○ Source failures
    - Information not available/not recorded so not presented at rounds
    - Relevant parties not all present at rounds
    - Notes/charts missing
    - Decisions from person leading rounds unclear
  - ○ Transmission failures
    - Information not passed on to relevant parties
    - No formal hand-off procedures
  - ○ Receiver failures
    - Instructions not followed

From: Nagpal, K., *et al.* (2012) Failures in communication and information transfer across the surgical care pathway: interview study. *BMJ Quality & Safety* **21**: 843–849. With permission of the publisher.

It is clear that multiple types of communication breakdown can occur at all stages of patient care, but one particular situation in patient care offers a greater opportunity for communication breakdown than most, that of patient hand-offs.

Patient hand-offs and transfers

Within the context of anesthesia, the entire perioperative period is vulnerable to communication breakdowns, with information loss occurring at every stage from the patient's first consultation, to care in the recovery room and ward area (Christian *et al.* 2006). But time points of particular concern are hand-offs of patients from caregiver to caregiver, and physical transfer of patients from one venue to another (see Chapter 8, "Structured communication: a beginning, middle, and an end" for additional discussion of patient hand-offs).

A hand-off occurs when there is a complete transfer of patient care from one person to another (e.g., from anesthetist to personnel in recovery or ICU) with the first person physically leaving the patient with the other.

A physical transfer in care is the physical movement of a patient from one location to another (e.g., moving from the CT imaging suite to the operating room). Transfers might or might not involve hand-offs, and vice versa (Greenberg *et al.* 2007). There are many consequences and costs of communication failure during hand-offs, including (Patterson & Woods 2001):

1 Creating an incorrect or incomplete model of the system's state.
2 Preventing the sharing of significant data or events.
3 Rendering caregivers unprepared to deal with consequences of previous events.
4 Caregivers are unable to anticipate future events.
5 Tasks cannot be performed for lack of knowledge necessary to perform the tasks.
6 Caregivers altering activities that are already in progress or that the team has agreed to do.
7 Creating an unwarranted shift in goals or plans.

Communication failures are distractions from doing a job well. As such they can cause stress and increase the likelihood that a caregiver will err in some aspect of patient care.

Distractions and stress

Distractions can cause stress, and stress plays a role in error generation. A bit of stress is not always bad of course; the often overgeneralized Yerkes–Dodson law outlines an inverted U-shaped relationship between arousal and learning (Yerkes & Dodson 1908). Performance may increase with increased arousal (physiological or mental stress), but only up to a point after which it can rapidly decline. It is likely the optimal state of arousal for any individual varies for both physical and mental stress, and depending on the task/activity being performed. As Leape has pointed out, a moderate level of stress yields the best performance, but poor performance and errors are more likely to occur at the extremes of boredom and panic (Leape 1994).

Under conditions of stress certain cognitive processes develop that lead to error generation, such as:

- **Coning of attention**—under the stress of an emergency there can be the tendency to concentrate on one piece of information to the exclusion of other pieces of information that may be germane to the problem at hand.
- **Reversion under stress**—recently learned behavior patterns are replaced by older, more familiar ones, even if they are inappropriate in the circumstances being encountered.

Pattern matching and biases

As previously stated, we humans prefer pattern matching to such a degree that Reason has stated, "[h]umans are furious pattern matchers" (Reason 2005), but sometimes the patterns do not match the situation. In discussing how the factors of self, context, and task are involved in making unsafe acts, Reason makes the analogy that they are "buckets of bad stuff," but that "full buckets" do not guarantee that an unsafe act will occur, nor that nearly empty ones will ensure safety because they are never wholly empty; rather it is probabilities that we are dealing with and not certainties (Reason 2004).

There are many habits of thought—biases—that alter the intuitive and analytical modes of thinking and lead to errors (Table 2.3). These biases and the intuitive and analytical modes of cognition are well suited for error analysis (Croskerry *et al.* 2013a, 2013b). The most important cognitive errors (biases) in anesthesia are: confirmation bias, premature closure, commission bias, sunk costs, anchoring, and omission bias (Table 2.4).

Individual responsibility within an organization

A good safety culture is one in which the organization promotes active awareness of the work environment and staff are encouraged to speak up and identify conditions and practices that might lead to an error or adverse incident. Of crucial importance, when staff do speak up they are treated fairly (see "Developing a safety culture" in Chapter 8) (Woodward 2005). What is the responsibility of the individual—the anesthetist—to the culture of safety and error prevention in such an organization? Individuals in complex organizations must be mindful, meaning that they perceive environmental elements within a volume of time and space and comprehend their meaning and project the status of those elements into the near future (Schulz *et al.* 2013). The individual maintains an adequate internal representation of the complex and dynamic environment and domains where time constants are short and conditions may change within seconds and minutes (Schulz *et al.* 2013). This said, a cautionary note is needed here. The flip side of mindfulness is not mindlessness. The usual scenario when one "loses mindfulness" is that something within the environment has captured the individual's attention and he or she is distracted from the task at hand.

Reason (2004) also discusses individual responsibility and refers to it as "mental preparedness," a state of mind wherein an individual:

- accepts that errors can and will occur;
- assesses the local "bad stuff" before embarking upon a task;
- has contingencies ready to deal with anticipated problems;
- is prepared to seek more qualified assistance;
- does not let professional courtesy get in the way of checking colleagues' knowledge and experience, particularly when they are strangers;
- appreciates that the path to adverse incidents is paved with false assumptions.

An anesthetist, of course, must be mindful when managing anesthesia so that dangerous conditions are anticipated, or recognized when they occur so that they can be promptly corrected (Gaba *et al.* 1994; Kurusz & Wheeldon 1990). Once a problem is recognized, its importance must be assessed and prioritized, for these steps determine how rapidly the problem needs to be addressed and how much additional verification is needed. During anesthesia of a patient with a specific

Table 2.3 Cognitive factors—biases—that influence decision-making and may lead to errors.

Aggregate bias—A clinician's belief that aggregated data do not apply to his or her patients because they are atypical or somehow exceptional; may lead to error of commission in that tests may be ordered which guidelines indicate are not required

Anchoring/fixation/"tunnel vision"—Focusing exclusively on a single feature of a case or an event to the exclusion of considering other aspects of the case. Includes **task fixation** wherein the clinician troubleshoots an alarm at the expense of situational awareness and attention to the patient

Ascertainment bias—When a clinician's thinking is shaped by prior expectation; gender bias and stereotyping are examples

Availability bias—The disposition to judge things as more likely or frequently occurring if they readily come to mind; choosing a diagnosis because it is at the forefront of a clinician's mind due to an emotionally charged memory of a bad experience

Bias blind spot—A flawed sense of invulnerability to bias

Commission bias—The tendency toward action rather than inaction even when those actions are not indicated or founded on desperation; stems from a sense of obligation to do good; it is more likely in overconfident clinicians

Confirmation bias—The tendency to only seek or see information that confirms or supports a diagnosis rather than look for information that refutes the diagnosis

Diagnosis momentum—Once a diagnosis is made it tends to stick with the patient such that what may have started as a possible diagnosis becomes definite and other possibilities are not considered

Feedback bias or sanction—When an error does not have immediate consequences such that considerable time elapses before the error is discovered and the absence of feedback is subconsciously processed as positive feedback. Croskerry calls this an ignorance trap that can occur in systems with poor feedback processes that prevent information getting to the decision maker (Croskerry 2003).

Fixation bias—persistent failure to revise a diagnosis or plan in the face of readily available evidence that suggests a revision is necessary

Framing effect—Allowing early presenting features to unduly influence decisions, particularly when transferring care from one clinician or team to another

Hindsight bias—Knowing the outcome may influence how one perceives and judges past events and thus prevent a realistic appraisal of what actually occurred

Omission bias—The tendency toward inaction rather than action out of fear of causing harm to a patient or to self by damaging professional reputation if wrong

Premature closure—Accepting a diagnosis before it has been fully verified

Sunk costs—The more effort and commitment invested in a plan, the harder it may become psychologically to abandon or revise that plan

Adapted from: Croskerry, P. (2003) *Academic Medicine* **78**(8): 775–780; Stiegler, M.P., *et al.* (2012) *British Journal of Anaesthesia* **108**(2): 229–235; Stiegler, M.P. & Tung. A. (2013) *Anesthesiology* **120**(1): 204–217.

condition, such as gastric dilatation volvulus, or one undergoing a specific surgical procedure, such as ovario-hysterectomy, anesthetists usually have a list of problems they expect to encounter and a subset of generic as well as specific solutions. Generic solutions usually gain the anesthetist additional time until a specific diagnosis is made and a solution can be implemented. However, additional errors may occur while a solution is being implemented, especially if the primary problem is not correctly identified. These errors can continue to generate new problems that also need resolution. Once an action has been taken the incident must be re-evaluated to determine whether the problem has been resolved or whether more action is needed to stabilize the patient. All this, of course, depends on the act of monitoring and using monitor-derived information.

Unfortunately, information provided by monitoring devices may be misleading because of artifacts,

transient physiological states (e.g., transient hypertension resulting from a transient supramaximal surgical stimulus such as traction on an ovary during ovariohysterectomy), misunderstanding how a particular monitor functions, or preconceptions of what to expect from a monitor. Furthermore, monitoring devices most commonly used in veterinary anesthesia are good for monitoring events involving the heart and lungs, but they do not specifically or directly monitor organs such as the liver or kidneys. For example, adverse effects of anesthesia on renal function will not be detected by monitors typically used to monitor anesthetized patients. It is only after the patient recovers, often several days after anesthesia, that renal problems, if present, become apparent. Of course, blood pressure monitoring may yield clues that the kidneys are at risk, especially if the patient is hypotensive, but this assumes a blood

Table 2.4 Cognitive errors (biases) considered to be the most important in anesthesia practice as identified by a survey of faculty, and the prevalence of those cognitive errors actually observed during clinical anesthesia.

Cognitive error	Faculty selection (%)	Order	Frequency observed (%)	Order
Anchoring	84.4	1	61.5	5
Availability bias	53.1	2	7.8	9
Premature closure	46.9	3	79.5	1
Confirmation bias	40.6	4	76.9	2
Framing effect	40.6	5	23.7	8
Commission bias	32.0	6	66.7	3
Overconfidence	32.0	7	53.8	7
Omission bias	28.1	8	61.5	6
Sunk costs	25.0	9	66.7	4

Data from: Stiegler, M.P., *et al*. (2012) Cognitive errors detected in anaesthesiology: a literature review and pilot study. *British Journal of Anaesthesia* **108**(2): 229–235. With permission of the publisher.

pressure monitor is being used and the information it yields is being acted upon.

Monitoring devices also may not be sensitive enough to detect a problem. A study designed to analyze human and technical factors contributing to anesthesia-associated complications yielded an important insight as to what monitored variables are pivotal in the early detection of critical incidents. Using breathing circuit disconnections during mechanical ventilation as an example of a critical incident, key events were identified that led to the initial discovery of the disconnection: change in pulse or arterial pressure (26%), directly observing the disconnect (24%), patient color (16%), a change in performance of the ventilator (13%), absent breath sounds (13%), absent chest movements (11%), poor [sic] arterial blood gases during routine sampling (5%), change in electrocardiogram (3%), and cardiac arrest (2%) (Newbower *et al*. 1981). Note that the ECG, a device frequently used and relied upon by veterinarians to monitor anesthetized patients, is an insensitive monitor for detecting this type of incident (airway disconnect) because it is not a specific monitor of the airway. One wonders if the results of this study, published in 1981, would have been different had pulse oximetry been used. Nonetheless, the mindful anesthetist is aware of the wealth of patient-related information that

monitoring devices provide, but is also aware of their limitations and traps.

Individuals in complex systems must consider standardizing procedures via checklists and guidelines as they can prevent errors and accidents (Heitmiller *et al*. 2007). Checklists may seem simplistic, but they have been found to significantly decrease morbidity and mortality in human patients (see "Checklists as error-reducing tools" in Chapter 8, for a fuller discussion of checklists) (Haynes *et al*. 2009). We contend that the same benefits accrue to veterinary medicine, specifically to anesthesia practice, but there are no studies to prove this contention. Checklists may be of a general nature, such as those routinely used to check out the integrity and functionality of anesthesia machines and ventilators prior to their use; or they may be more specific for managing a patient undergoing a specific type of procedure. Some believe that standard operating procedures (SOPs) and checklists limit an anesthetist's options for developing protocols for individual patients, but this misses the purpose of these tools: they are designed to "jog" one's memory so that key elements essential to good patient management are not overlooked (error of omission) during the "doing" of anesthesia. They are meant to trigger and assist analytical modes of problem-solving, not distract the anesthetist from them.

Error causation: other factors

As shown in Figure 2.1, the environment within which we work is not confined to the surgical theater, imaging suite, or examination room, but is influenced by outside factors, many of which, although beyond our control, can cause harm either to the patient or to those working with the patient. For example, difficult clients may distract us from the tasks at hand, or unavailability of drugs or supplies that are used in daily practice can adversely affect a practice. Financial constraints may make clinicians cut corners in diagnostic and treatment pathways, which, although well-meaning, can lead to significant errors in patient management. A vicious dog is its own worst enemy in terms of receiving optimal care; often times shortcuts must be taken for reasons of safety both for those working with the animal and the animal itself. Such shortcuts can lead to errors.

Conclusion

Errors can be reduced through a number of strategies, including (Leape 1994):

- Recognizing that all factors—technical, organizational, human, and other factors—must be considered when striving to prevent and manage errors. Focusing only on human factors is counterproductive and will not lessen the incidence of errors.
- Fostering an environment that is open, willing, and able to learn from errors is a crucial feature of the learning or high reliability organization.
- Improving communication through the awareness of factors that contribute to communication breakdowns and failures, and by facilitating access to information, both patient-related information and information highlighting errors and near misses when they occur.
- Recognizing that in complex, dynamic systems checklists can reduce the risk of making errors by jogging one's memory so that key elements essential to good patient management are not overlooked.

We now turn our attention to strategies for reporting and analyzing patient safety incidents.

References

Allnutt, M.F. (1987) Human factors in accidents. *British Journal of Anaesthesia* **59**(7): 856–864.

Battles, J.B. & Shea, C.E. (2001) A system of analyzing medical errors to improve GME curricula and programs. *Academic Medicine* **76**(2): 125–133.

Christian, C.K., *et al.* (2006) A prospective study of patient safety in the operating room. *Surgery* **139**(2): 159–173.

Croskerry, P. (2003) The importance of cognitive errors in diagnosis and strategies to minimize them. *Academic Medicine* **78**(8): 775–780.

Croskerry, P., *et al.* (2013a) Cognitive debiasing 1: Origins of bias and theory of debiasing. *BMJ Quality & Safety* **22**(Suppl. 2): ii58–ii64.

Croskerry, P., *et al.* (2013b) Cognitive debiasing 2: Impediments to and strategies for change. *BMJ Quality & Safety* **22**(Suppl. 2): ii65–ii72.

Diller, T., *et al.* (2014) The human factors analysis classification system (HFACS) applied to health care. *American Journal of Medical Quality* **29**(3): 181–190.

Gaba, D.M., Fish, K.J., & Howard, S.K. (1994) *Crisis Management in Anesthesiology*. Philadelphia: Churchill Livingstone.

Garnerin, P., *et al.* (2002) Root-cause analysis of an airway filter occlusion: A way to improve the reliability of the respiratory circuit. *British Journal of Anaesthesia* **89**(4): 633–635.

Garnerin, P., *et al.* (2006) Using system analysis to build a safety culture: Improving the reliability of epidural analgesia. *Acta Anaesthesiologica Scandinavica* **50**(9): 1114–1119.

Greenberg, C.C., *et al.* (2007) Patterns of communication breakdowns resulting in injury to surgical patients. *Journal of the American College of Surgeons* **204**(4): 533–540.

Haerkens, M.H., *et al.* (2015) Crew resource management in the intensive care unit: A prospective 3-year cohort study. *Acta Anaesthesiologica Scandinavica* **59**(10): 1319–1329.

Hall, K.H. (2002) Reviewing intuitive decision-making and uncertainty: The implications for medical education. *Medical Education* **36**(3): 216–224.

Haynes, A.B., *et al.* (2009) A surgical safety checklist to reduce morbidity and mortality in a global population. *New England Journal of Medicine* **360**(5): 491–499.

Heitmiller, E., *et al.* (2007) Identifying and learning from mistakes. *Anesthesiology* **106**(4): 654–656.

Helmreich, R.L. (2000) On error management: Lessons from aviation. *British Medical Journal* **320**(7237): 781–785.

Hofmeister, E.H., *et al.* (2014) Development, implementation and impact of simple patient safety interventions in a university teaching hospital. *Veterinary Anaesthesia & Analgesia*, **41**(3): 243–248.

Hollnagel, E. (2009) *The ETTO Principle: Efficiency-Thoroughness Trade-Off: Why Things that Go Right Sometimes Go Wrong.* Aldershot, UK: Ashgate.

Karsh, B.T., *et al.* (2006) A human factors engineering paradigm for patient safety: Designing to support the performance of the healthcare professional. *Quality and Safety in Health Care* **15**(Suppl. 1): i59–i65.

Klemola, U.M. (2000) The psychology of human error revisited. *European Journal of Anaesthesiology* **17**(6): 401–401.

Kohn, L.T., Corrigan, J.M., & Donaldson, M.S. (eds) (2000) *To Err is Human: Building a Safer Health System.* Washington, DC: National Academy Press.

Kovacs, G. & Croskerry, P. (1999) Clinical decision making: An emergency medicine perspective. *Academic Emergency Medicine* **6**(9): 947–952.

Kruskal, J.B., *et al.* (2008) Managing an acute adverse event in a radiology department. *Radiographics* **28**(5): 1237–1250.

Kurusz, M. & Wheeldon, D.R. (1990) Risk containment during cardiopulmonary bypass. *Seminars in Thoracic and Cardiovascular Surgery* **2**: 400–409.

Leape, L.L. (1994) Error in medicine. *Journal of the American Medical Association* **272**(23): 1851–1857.

Leape, L.L. (2002) Reporting of adverse events. *New England Journal of Medicine* **347**(20): 1633–1638.

Lingard, L., *et al.* (2004) Communication failures in the operating room: An observational classification of recurrent types and effects. *Quality & Safety in Health Care* **13**(5): 330–334.

McLaughlin, K., *et al.* (2014) Reexamining our bias against heuristics. *Advances in Health Sciences Education: Theory and Practice* **19**(3): 457–464.

Nagpal, K., *et al.* (2012) Failures in communication and information transfer across the surgical care pathway: Interview study. *BMJ Quality & Safety* **21**(10): 843–849.

Newbower, R.S., *et al.* (1981) Learning from anesthesia mishaps: Analysis of critical incidents in anesthesia helps reduce patient risk. *QRB Quality Review Bulletin* **7**(3): 10–16.

Palazzolo, C. & Stoutenburgh, G. (1997) Turning a veterinary hospital into a learning organization. *Journal of the American Veterinary Medical Association* **210**(3): 337–339.

Patterson, E.S. & Woods, D. (2001) Shift changes, updates, and the on-call architecture in space shuttle mission control. *Computer Supported Cooperative Work (CSCW)* **10**(3–4): 317–346.

Reason, J.T. (1990a) *Human Error.* Cambridge: Cambridge University Press.

Reason, J.T. (1990b) The contribution of latent human failures to the breakdown of complex systems. *Philosophical Transactions of the Royal Society of London. Series B, Biological Sciences* **327**(1241): 475–484.

Reason, J.T. (2000) Safety paradoxes and safety culture. *Injury Control and Safety Promotion* **7**(1): 3–14.

Reason, J.T. (2004) Beyond the organisational accident: The need for "error wisdom" on the frontline. *Quality and Safety in Health Care,* **13**(Suppl. 2): ii28–ii33.

Reason, J.T. (2005) Safety in the operating theatre – part 2: Human error and organisational failure. *Quality & Safety in Health Care* **14**(1): 56–60.

Reason, J.T. (2008) *The Human Contribution: Unsafe Acts, Accidents, and Heroic Recoveries.* Burlington, VT: Ashgate Publishing Co.

Reason, J.T., *et al.* (2001) Diagnosing "vulnerable system syndrome": An essential prerequisite to effective risk management. *Quality in Health Care* **10**(Suppl. 2): ii21–ii25.

Schulz, C.M., *et al.* (2013) Situation awareness in anesthesia: Concept and research. *Anesthesiology* **118**(3): 729–742.

Stanovich, K.E. (2011) *Rationality and the Reflective Mind.* New York: Oxford University Press.

Stiegler, M.P. & Tung, A. (2014) Cognitive processes in anesthesiology decision making. *Anesthesiology* **120**(1): 204–217.

Stiegler, M.P., *et al.* (2012) Cognitive errors detected in anaesthesiology: A literature review and pilot study. *British Journal of Anaesthesia* **108**(2): 229–235.

Sutcliffe, K.M. (2011) High reliability organizations (HROs). *Best Practice & Research in Clinical Anaesthesiology* **25**(2): 133–144.

Vincent, C., *et al.* (1998) Framework for analysing risk and safety in clinical medicine. *British Medical Journal* **316**(7138): 1154–1157.

Vincent, C., *et al.* (2014) Safety measurement and monitoring in healthcare: A framework to guide clinical teams and healthcare organisations in maintaining safety. *BMJ Quality & Safety* **23**(8): 670–677.

Vogus, T.J. & Hilligoss, B. (2015) The underappreciated role of habit in highly reliable healthcare. *BMJ Quality & Safety* doi:10.1136/bmjqs-2015-004512.

Wald, H. & Shojania, K.G. (2001) Incident reporting. In: *Making Health Care Safer: A Critical Analysis of Patient Safety Practices* (eds K.G. Shojania, B.W. Duncan, K.M. McDonald, & R.M. Wachter). Rockville, MD: Agency for Healthcare Research and Quality, pp. 41–50.

Weick, K.E. (2002) The reduction of medical errors through mindful interdependence. In: *Medical Errors: What Do We Know? What Do We Do?* (eds M.M. Rosenthal & K.M. Sutcliffe), 1st edn. San Francisco, CA: Jossey-Bass, pp. 177–199.

Welch, S.J., *et al.* (2013) Strategies for improving communication in the emergency department: Mediums and messages in a noisy environment. *Journal on Quality and Patient Safety* **39**(6): 279–286.

Wheeler, S.J. & Wheeler, D.W. (2005) Medication errors in anaesthesia and critical care. *Anaesthesia* **60**(3): 257–273.

Woodward, S.J. (2005) Will the future continue to repeat the past? *Quality and Safety in Health Care* **14**(2): 74.

Yerkes, R.M. & Dodson, J.D. (1908) The relation of strength of stimulus to rapidity of habit-formation. *Journal of Comparative Neurology and Psychology,* **18**: 459–482.

CHAPTER 3

Reporting and Analyzing Patient Safety Incidents

The Universe is made of stories, not of atoms.
  Muriel Rukeyser, The Speed of Darkness (1968)

Incident analysis, properly understood, is not a retrospective search for root causes but an attempt to look to the future. In a sense, the particular causes of the incident in question do not matter as they are now in the past. However, the weaknesses of the system revealed are still present and could lead to the next incident.
  C.A. Vincent (2004)

To act you have to know—In medicine, both human and veterinary, there is a culture of infallibility, one in which mistakes are unacceptable and made only by bad clinicians. After all, it is difficult to accept an error when a life has been lost or a patient harmed. An effect of this cultural mindset is that error is under-reported and remains an under-recognized and hidden problem. In fact, discussion of error is actively avoided, generally considered taboo and unthinkable, despite the fact that errors occur regularly and will continue to occur.

It has been estimated that as many as 400,000 patients die prematurely in the United States as a result of hospital-associated preventable harm (James 2013), and it has been estimated that preventable errors occur in up to 7.2% of hospitalized patients (Baker *et al.* 2004; Hogan *et al.* 2012; Kennerly *et al.* 2014). It seems naively improbable, verging on arrogance, to think that a lower error rate exists in veterinary medicine. The problem is that we just don't know. In human medicine we are aware of the tip of the iceberg in terms of the impact of errors on patients, while in veterinary medicine we're sailing along seemingly ignoring the fact that icebergs even exist.

So it is safe to say that we are far behind human medicine and anesthesia when it comes to recognizing and managing error. We have even further to go before we can label veterinary anesthesia as being safe, before we can state with confidence that the risk of anesthesia causing preventable and unnecessary harm to our patients is negligible. Our first step is to recognize and accept that errors occur in veterinary medicine and that all of our practices can be made safer. The next task is for us to establish the extent and nature of the problem by discovering what errors occur, how often, and their true causality. This means we must make an effort to start reporting, analyzing, sharing, and discussing the errors we encounter. At first glance we may consider errors to be mundane, small events without consequence to our patients. But when error-prone conditions or events become aligned the errors that occur can have significant adverse impact on patient safety. For this reason we must view each error as a learning opportunity in our efforts to promote patient safety. Reporting and analyzing even basic errors can cause "Eureka!" moments that accelerate learning, understanding, and self-awareness, and give invaluable insight into the systems and processes with which we are involved on a daily basis (Tripp 1993). These insights can be significant catalysts in the process of change (Cope & Watts 2000).

The limitation in only counting errors

Highlighting only the occurrence and frequency of errors, such as using a simple error log, can be useful in some circumstances and may present opportunities for obvious, simple interventions. But there can be shortcomings. For example, at a large teaching hospital,

Errors in Veterinary Anesthesia, First Edition. John W. Ludders and Matthew McMillan.
© 2017 John Wiley & Sons, Inc. Published 2017 by John Wiley & Sons, Inc.

operating room staff members voluntarily reported errors on a simple log when errors occurred (Hofmeister *et al.* 2014). After a period of 11½ months the log was analyzed and 20 incidences of the pop-off valve being accidentally left closed when setting up the operating room, 16 incidences of temporarily unrecognized esophageal intubation, five incidences of accidental intra-arterial drug administration, and 20 other medication errors were recorded. This is the first time such data have been collected and reported in the veterinary anesthesia literature; it is likely that this frequency of error events is mirrored in veterinary teaching hospitals throughout the world.

As a result of the initial findings, specific checks ("Technician checked OR" and "Technician Confirmed Intubation") were incorporated into the anesthetic process. In addition, a different color for bandages covering arterial catheters was instituted, and a standard operating procedure (SOP) was created that required patient name, drug name, and route of administration be read aloud prior to administering any drug to an anesthetized patient. Gratifyingly, these interventions led to a 75% reduction in the incidence of pop-off valves being left closed, a 75% reduction in unrecognized esophageal intubation, a 60% decrease in accidental intra-arterial injection, and a 50% decrease in medication error. Case closed! Or is it? Could more be learned about these errors? Surely a reduction to zero should be what we strive for?

This was obviously a relatively successful outcome based on simple and efficient solutions, but perhaps this approach oversimplified the errors. Superficial analysis of incidents often uncovers only a single source of human error, which in turn often leads to blaming only the fallible individual while failing to recognize that we are all fallible; this approach also ignores the role of the system in the error. This leaves a lot of potentially vital information regarding error causality hidden and not analyzed. For example, assuming that pop-off valves were left shut merely due to human failing (be it lack of concentration, forgetfulness, distractions, etc.) fails to recognize something that has already been established: errors are often rooted in latent conditions within the system.

So, what if we ask: why did this human failing occur? What were the conditions that allowed these errors to occur? Could this approach identify other potential contributing factors? The answer is most definitely yes.

You could ask, does this matter in this case? No harm came to any patients and seemingly effective barriers against the errors are now in place. Perhaps it does matter, but we won't know unless we fully analyze the errors and their underlying causes. Perhaps the technicians responsible for setting up the breathing systems in the operating room felt rushed due to the service being understaffed or having been assigned too many tasks and responsibilities. Was there a failure in training? Was there a larger problem in that the entire anesthetic machine in the operating room was not being fully checked (not just the pop-off valves)? The superficial analysis may have worked well to prevent the specific errors that were identified, but the underlying latent factors causing the errors in the first place still persist and, under different circumstances, will cause errors of a different nature. For example, if the anesthetic machines are not thoroughly checked then one day an empty auxiliary oxygen cylinder might go unnoticed and leave a patient without oxygen if the oxygen pipeline supply fails. Alternatively, further analysis might have identified why veterinary students had difficulty correctly intubating patients, a finding that could have led to a solution that more fully addressed the problem of failed intubations such as simulator training.

How can we learn the most from our errors?

An error report requires a thorough analysis in order to uncover the factors that detract from effective task performance, to find latent factors—underlying root causes—that created the environment in which the error could occur, factors that might have been responsible for impairing the performance level of the individual. Appropriate analysis helps to discover not only what occurred but also why it occurred. Merely tallying up the number of specific errors, for example, through using an error log, and then responding to them is insufficient; instead we need to analyze errors and the circumstances surrounding them. To do this we need to stop thinking of an error as a single event, but as an "incident." Viewing an error as an incident moves away from the idea that it is a single, spontaneously occurring event and moves toward the view that it is the manifestation of a series of events and latent conditions that have evolved over time under a set of circumstances in a specific environment. Viewing an error as an incident—a chain of events—means that we have to create a far more complex account of errors; the most natural of these accounts is the "error narrative."

The importance of narrative

A narrative is an account of events (an incident or story) over time; it involves relating people with the places, objects, and actions involved in an incident, but also recounts their reasoning, feelings, beliefs, and theories at the time of the incident, albeit often retrospectively. A good narrative report should provide the context to the incident described (basically who, what, where, when, and how) thus allowing a reader or listener to hypothesize regarding the reasons why the incident happened. As such a narrative is more than a factual list of physical events; it outlines both cause(s) and effect(s) and also provides a psychological overview of those who were involved. Developing a narrative is a natural form of human communication, one from which we learn well, perhaps more so than from other modes of learning, such as logical-scientific communication or deductive reasoning (Betsch *et al.* 2011; Dahlstrom 2014; Winterbottom *et al.* 2008). But why? Surely we can learn all we need to know from a listing of the facts of the incident that occurred? Well, no! As already discussed it's not just about the events, but also about the human factors involved in an incident, those factors that affected the cognitive and physical performance of those involved, the entirety of the context within which the incident occurred. This is much more complex and requires more thought and processing. So why does a narrative help?

Narrative has been demonstrated to be an effective tool for understanding and learning because it allows more complex cognitive processing. This depth of cognitive processing has been attributed to two properties (Gerrig 1993): (1) transportation of the reader or listener to another time and place in a manner that is so compelling it appears real; (2) the reader or listener performs the narrative in their mind, lives the experience by drawing inferences, and experiences through empathy. This has been shown experimentally using functional magnetic resonance imaging (fMRI) to map the brain activity of storytellers and listeners (Stephens *et al.* 2010). During narrative storytelling the listener's brain activity is coupled spatially and temporally, albeit with a small delay, with the speaker's narrative. This

phenomenon—"speaker-listener neural coupling"—may be a fundamental method the brain utilizes to convey information, make meaning of the information, and bring understanding of the world (Wells 1986). In the field of patient safety a rich narrative report is considered the only method capable of providing a full enough account of an incident to allow the complex conditions and processes that contributed to the event to be properly communicated and analyzed (Cook *et al.* 1998).

There are several methods by which a narrative report can be made. The most common are open discussions in the form of focus groups (such as morbidity and mortality rounds—M&Ms), interview techniques (including critical incident technique—CITs), and voluntary reporting.

Focus groups: morbidity and mortality rounds (M&Ms)

Although not an incident reporting and analysis method, morbidity and mortality rounds can be a useful starting point for identifying and combating error within a hospital or practice. These rounds are focus groups brought together following an incident of patient morbidity or mortality, and are generally used as part of a practice's clinical audit and governance process. As such they are a means for promoting transparency concerning an organization's safety climate and for raising everyone's awareness of patient safety through open discussions on patient management and safety issues. They may be convened after specific incidents, or may recur on a scheduled basis.

The goal is to promote dialogue as to what went well and what did not, and what could be done differently on a specific case or set of cases involving errors or adverse outcomes. Unfortunately, morbidity and mortality rounds are usually only performed when a patient suffers serious harm or when there is an internal or external complaint made regarding management of a patient. In these situations case analysis can become a superficial process and a forum for criticism, a finger-pointing exercise with simplistic answers that often focus only on the person at the "sharp end." Unfortunately, once blame is apportioned and simple remedial action is taken, the analysis stops and the system goes on as usual.

However, when performed well, discussions often highlight failings within systems as well as information on how overall case management could be improved.

Cases are best presented following the timeline that they traveled through the hospital. It should be ensured that every member of staff involved with the case is able to describe their involvement, giving their interpretation of the events surrounding the case. An error or adverse incident should be considered an emotional event for the people involved and handled accordingly. Intense feelings such as anger, regret, frustration, helplessness, embarrassment, and guilt can be triggered in those involved. These emotions can be externalized in a variety of manners leading to an emotionally charged discussion (Cope & Watts 2000). For these reasons all enquiries and dialogue should be performed respectfully and empathetically, mindful of the sensibilities of those involved.

The case description should be followed by a reflective discussion, open to input from the floor. This allows a multifaceted interpretation of the events surrounding the case. Some method for allowing input from all who wish to be heard is required as too often it is the more senior and vocal members of the team who get their opinions heard, with the more junior members being left as non-participatory observers. For these sessions to be successful proper leadership and a neutral, non-confrontational, non-judgmental approach is required. The leadership role ideally should be provided by someone respected by all parties involved in the case, one who is generally considered to be fair, calm, and unbiased during conflict. The discussion moderator should be willing to step in and redirect discussions when they digress, become accusatory, or aggressive.

When managed well, morbidity and mortality rounds are recognized as being an important platform to explore, disseminate, and address in a timely manner system issues that contribute to errors and adverse incidents. However, many participants may be unwilling to share their thoughts in such an open forum. In such situations private interviews may be more appropriate.

Interview techniques

Private interview techniques are an alternative approach to morbidity and mortality rounds. In general, a senior staff member informally discusses the incident with each individual member of the team involved with the case. This approach avoids individuals feeling the pressure of having an audience of peers listening to their successes and failings, and is one that encourages a more honest and less defensive appraisal of the incident.

However, private interviews reduce the learning experience for the rest of the team. Sometimes individuals feel more threatened and intimidated when separated from the team and as a result feel less empowered to speak freely as they no longer have the support of their peers.

Another problem is that interviews may be biased by the interviewer's point of view, a bias that may direct the interview along a specific path. For this method to work successfully this type of analysis is better performed as part of a more structured interview such as the critical incident technique.

Critical incident technique (CIT)

The critical incident technique is a qualitative research method with its origins in job analysis as performed by industrial and organizational psychologists. It sets out to solve practical problems using broad psychological principles. The technique is based on firsthand reports of the incident, including the manner and environment in which the task was executed. Information is traditionally gathered in face-to-face interviews. During an interview, respondents are simply asked to recall specific events from their own perspective, using their own terms and language. Questions such as: "What happened during the event, including what led up to it and what followed it?", "What did they do?", and "Tell me what you were thinking at the time" are typically used to start the interview. As such the critical incident technique is not constrained by direct questioning or preconceptions of what factors in the incident were important to the respondent. As a result the interviewee is free to give a full range of responses without bias being introduced by the interviewer.

Introduced in 1954 by John C. Flanagan (1954), the critical incident technique actually had its roots in aviation during World War II when procedures for selecting pilots were investigated, specifically seeking why pilot candidates failed to learn to fly. Findings revealed that all too often analyses of pilot candidates were based on clichés and stereotypes such as "poor judgment," or "lack of inherent ability" and "unsuitable temperament" (Flanagan 1954), but other specific behaviors were consistently reported and became the basis for ongoing research into pilot candidate selection. This research led to better methods for collecting data and became "the first large scale systematic attempt to gather specific incidents of effective or ineffective behavior with respect to a designated activity" (Flanagan 1954).

After the war, some of the psychologists involved in that program established the American Institute for Research (AIR) with the aim of systematically studying human behavior (Flanagan 1954). It was through the Institute that Flanagan formally developed the CIT. It was used initially in aviation to determine critical requirements for the work of United States Air Force officers and commercial airline pilots. Subsequently, the critical incident technique was expanded to establish critical requirements for naval research personnel, air traffic controllers, workers at General Motors Corporation, and even dentistry (Flanagan 1954). The latter, although not generally recognized as such at the time, was probably the first application of this technique in a medical discipline.

When Flanagan introduced this technique he stated that it "was...very effective in obtaining information from individuals concerning their own errors, from subordinates concerning errors of their superiors, from supervisors with respect to their subordinates, and also from participants with respect to co-participants" (Flanagan 1954).

Critical incident technique in anesthesia

The first documented suggestion to apply the critical incident technique to the practice of anesthesia was made in 1971 by Blum in a letter to the journal *Anesthesiology* (Blum 1971). Blum suggested the need to apply human factors and ergonomic principles when designing anesthetic equipment because human perception and reaction can influence the effectiveness of the "man-machine system."

In 1978, Cooper reported the results of a modified critical incident technique, what he called a critical incident analysis, to perform a retrospective analysis of human error and equipment failure in anesthesia (Cooper *et al.* 1978). Information was obtained by interviewing anesthesiologists and asking them to describe preventable incidents they had observed or participated in that involved either a human error or equipment malfunction. Critical incidents were defined when an event fulfilled the following four criteria:

1 It involved an error by a team member or a malfunctioning piece of equipment.
2 The patient was under the care of an anesthetist.
3 It could be described in detail by someone who was involved with or observed the incident.
4 It was clearly preventable.

Table 3.1 Twenty-three major categories of information derived through interviews with anesthesiologists who had observed or participated in preventable incidents involving either human error or equipment malfunction.

Major categories of information	
1 Error or failure	13 Secondary consequence to
2 Location of incident	patient
3 Date of incident	14 Who discovered incident
4 Time of day	15 Who discovered incident cause
5 Hospital location	16 Discovery delay
6 Patient condition before	17 Correction delay
the incident	18 Discovery of cause of delay
7 OR scheduling	19 Individual responsible for
8 Length of OR procedure	incident
9 OR procedure	20 Involvement of interviewee
10 Anesthetic technique	21 Interviewee experience at
11 Associated factors	time of interview
12 Immediate consequence	22 Related incidents
to patient	23 Important side comments

From Cooper, J.B., *et al.* (1978) Preventable anesthesia mishaps: a study of human factors. *Anesthesiology* 49: 399–406. With permission of the publisher.

The interviewers were allowed to elicit details of the event through the use of generalized, prompting questions where needed, but they were not allowed to suggest any particular occurrence. Information was captured and organized into 23 categories (Table 3.1) (Cooper *et al.* 1978).

The results gave a fascinating insight into an area of anesthesia that until then had remained unexplored. Cooper found that human error was involved in 82% of the preventable incidents while equipment failure was involved in only 14% of the incidents. Forty-four different predisposing factors were identified (the most common are listed in Table 3.2), including haste, fatigue and distraction, poor labeling of drugs, inadequate supervision, and poor communication.

This study is recognized as being innovative in medicine and pivotal in driving forward the patient safety movement in anesthesia (Cullen *et al.* 2000), and did so long before the publication of the Institute of Medicine's "To Err is Human" report in 2000. In fact the methods and results reported are still relevant and have become the basis of incident reporting systems in anesthesia today.

Table 3.2 The most common predisposing factors for errors in anesthesia in order of reported frequency (count; % frequency rounded to whole number).

Categories of information	
1 Inadequate total experience (77; 16%)	15 Distraction (13; 3%)
2 Inadequate familiarity with equipment/device (45; 9%)	16 Poor labeling of controls, drugs, etc. (12; 2%)
3 Poor communication with team, lab, etc. (27; 6%)	17 Supervision—other factors (12; 2%)
4 Haste (26; 5%)	18 Situation precluded normal precautions (10; 2%)
5 Inattention/carelessness (26; 5%)	19 Inadequate familiarity with anesthetic technique (10; 2%)
6 Fatigue (24; 5%)	20 Teaching activity under way (9; 2%)
7 Excessive dependency on other personnel (24; 5%)	21 Apprehension (8; 2%)
8 Failure to perform a normal check (22; 5%)	22 Emergency case (6; 1%)
9 Training or experience including other factors (22; 5%)	23 Demanding or difficult case (6; 1%)
10 Supervisor not present enough (18; 4%)	24 Boredom (5; 1%)
11 Environment or colleagues—other factors (18; 4%)	25 Nature of activity—other factors (5; 1%)
12 Visual field restricted (17; 4%)	26 Insufficient preparation (3; 1%)
13 Mental or physical including other factors (16; 3%)	27 Slow procedure (3; 1%)
14 Inadequate familiarity with surgical procedure (14; 3%)	28 Other (3; 1%)

From Cooper, J.B., *et al.* (1978) Preventable anesthesia mishaps: a study of human factors. *Anesthesiology* 49: 399–406. With permission of the publisher.

Voluntary reporting systems

Voluntary reporting systems are the most commonly used method in human medicine for error and patient safety incident analysis. When analyzed and managed properly voluntary reports are considered an effective method for inducing behavioral change in healthcare teams (Garrouste-Orgeas *et al.* 2012).

A number of vital components make up a good voluntary report (see Table 3.3). Probably the most important factor is a free text section in which the reporter outlines a narrative chain of events. An effective error reporting system encourages the reporter to provide a comprehensive and structured narrative that facilitates later analysis and investigations. This narrative should form a detailed description of what occurred and how it deviated significantly, either positively or negatively, from what is normal or expected (Edvardsson 1992).

The primary aim of the narrative is to fully define the incident so that it can be fully and properly analyzed. Reporters should be encouraged to reflect critically upon the incident, questioning the actions and involvement of all the individuals involved, alongside the local practices, processes, and procedures (Tripp 1993). Reporters should be asked to identify critical requirements for success that were not carried out and the reasons behind these omissions. These reasons should include the attitudes, behaviors, knowledge, or skills of those individuals involved; the work environment; any problems with teamwork or communication as well as any actions and inactions that occurred. As a consequence, the perceptions and awareness of the reporter are an important aspect of this section and the structure of the report should not influence, lead, or bias the reporter. The report should seek to gather information in the same manner as that used in the critical incident technique. A report should also be used to gather other background information about the incident that lends itself to the analytical framework used to analyze the incident. The type of background data commonly collected alongside the narrative report include:

- Location where the incident occurred.
- Timing of the incident (date and time).
- Information about the person reporting (e.g., their profession and role in the healthcare system).
- Any actions taken as a result of the incident.
- Patient outcome.
- Patient details.
- Mitigating circumstances.
- More specific enquiries about the root causes.

Online electronic reporting systems are becoming available and have the advantage of being more

Table 3.3 Characteristics necessary for an effective web-based voluntary reporting system, characteristics that help ensure incidents are reported appropriately.

• Easy to find and widely accessible
  ○ One button access from local systems
  ○ Common website address for national systems
  ○ Links from all hospital computers
  ○ Accessible from home
• Easy to enter case information
  ○ Simplicity
  ○ Pre-populated patient data
  ○ Intuitive flow of data entry
  ○ Menu driven
  ○ Checkbox data entry
  ○ Reactive logic, to hide irrelevant fields
  ○ Single narrative text box
  ○ No mandatory elements
• Data elements and definitions created by consensus process
	• Assured confidentiality
	  ○ Legal disclaimer at front
	  ○ Transparency about who will see report
	• Anonymous data entry
	  ○ Collection into appropriately structured database
	  ○ Transparent schema allowing sorting under multiple classification systems
	  ○ Search capability for finding and reviewing free text items
	• Visible use of data to improve patient safety
	  ○ Publication of de-identified case reports and narratives
	  ○ Publication of aggregated reports and trends
	  ○ Sharing of aggregate data with outside stakeholder

From: Dutton, R.P. (2014) Improving safety through incident reporting. *Current Anesthesiology Reports* 4: 84–89. With permission of the publisher.

accessible to individuals wishing to report an incident. Notable electronic reporting systems include the Anesthesia Incident Reporting System (AIRS) developed by the Anesthesia Quality Institute (AQI), a federally designated patient safety organization. Both an online report form and a smartphone application are available. Reports submitted through the Anesthesia Incident Reporting System are uploaded securely onto the Anesthesia Quality Institute's server, where they can be analyzed (https://www.aqihq.org/airs/airsIntro.aspx). Table 3.3 lists characteristics necessary for an effective web-based voluntary reporting system (Dutton 2014).

The most important and well-recognized characteristics of successful reporting systems are provision of a non-punitive environment, assurance of confidentiality, and submission of reports to an independent body that provides expert analysis and feedback to the person who submitted the report.

A non-punitive environment

The most difficult characteristic to create is that of a non-punitive environment, one that encourages reporting and admitting errors by ensuring that those involved are not punished as a result of submitting the report. To achieve this at all levels of veterinary medicine will involve a cultural change, a paradigm shift from a blame culture to a just culture (one that does not hold people culpable for making honest mistakes, but which

penalizes neglectful behavior and misconduct). Each of us needs to admit that we make errors and that things go wrong, admissions made not only to ourselves but to our peers and juniors. This evolution will only be successful if this filters from the top downwards, if those in the higher echelons of their respective practices, specialties, and organizations openly discuss their failures and errors alongside their successes. Whatever other changes are put in place, success in improving patient safety depends on this leadership from above. But one aspect of reporting errors that probably offsets any shortcomings in leadership is to ensure that all reports remain confidential.

Confidentiality

If healthcare professionals are to voluntarily report safety incidents and error, then they must know that there will be no personal or professional consequences for their candor. After all, as Cooper asked, "why should we expect clinicians to report their own adverse outcomes if reporting might jeopardize their career?" (Cooper 1996). The identity of the reporter, organization or practice, and patient should be protected by some sort of organizational or legal arrangement that ensures confidentiality. Some reporting systems go further than this, with reports being anonymous in nature. Anonymity gives an extra level of reassurance to further allay the fear of repercussions to those submitting the reports. However, anonymity also has at least two drawbacks. Firstly, the system can become a bulletin board for problems and issues that staff may have regarding their jobs. This background noise of discontent might hide the potentially vital signal of a critical safety report. This type of interference becomes particularly problematic where there is little constructive communication between frontline workers and their supervisors. Secondly, and probably of more importance, is that anonymity makes it impossible for those analyzing the report to gain further clarification from those who made the report or where data may not be complete for some incidents thus limiting proper and full analysis. Although confidentiality is a fundamental aspect of a successful reporting system, providing anonymity as an important element potentially limits the usefulness of reports.

Reporting to an independent third party

Using a respected independent third party to collect and analyze reported data is a useful and effective principle (Billings 1998). This community approach to data collection and analysis offers the reporter reassurance that the data will be analyzed away from his or her workplace by a person who is not a direct superior. The independent third party acts as a "firewall," an additional layer of separation between the reporter and potential consequences. An additional benefit of having data compiled by an independent third party is that the data will be shared and disseminated to a wider audience thus maximizing the impact of any critical information.

Expert analysis

For a report to achieve its full potential as a learning opportunity and tool for change it must be analyzed appropriately. Reports must be analyzed by experienced individuals who understand human factors and systems approaches to problem-solving. A good working knowledge of the specific clinical environments under evaluation and the nuances of the specialties under scrutiny is essential. Merely collecting and collating data will have little impact, so a network of expert analysts will be required if any large-scale reporting system is to succeed.

Feedback

Reporting will be encouraged if those submitting reports believe that the data are being used effectively. The only way to achieve this is by providing appropriate feedback

to the reporter. One method is to give the reporter the option of receiving an expert analysis and opinion of each case they report. This individual feedback helps reinforce the learning opportunities for the individual, in essence giving them a "return" for making their report. Furthermore, this feedback provides a strong potential for learning. As Gene Rochlin at the University of California-Berkley wrote, "[h]uman learning takes place through action. Trial-and-error defines limits, but its complement, trial and success...builds judgment and confidence. To not be allowed to err is not to be allowed to learn" (Rochlin 2012). A second commonly employed method is use of a regular newsletter that outlines important findings, statistics, and improvements gathered over a given time period. These newsletters can also include anonymized individual reports, analyses, and editorials to highlight specific safety concerns. A third approach, that of safety bulletins, can be employed to facilitate rapid and immediate dissemination of important safety concerns; these can be in the form of email alerts or notices on websites. Finally, an active contribution to academic literature in the form of epidemiological papers and scientific publications will help to cement reporting error into the consciousness of the profession.

Limitations of voluntary reporting

There are a number of limitations that must be considered before a voluntary reporting system can be implemented successfully. For example, incident reports can be too brief, fragmented, muddled, and biased by the reporter's personal view of events. To overcome these shortcomings multiple reports from different viewpoints are collected and used to analyze an incident. Voluntary reports also generally underestimate the number of errors and incidents that occur. A number of factors can account for this: reporting can be time consuming for the individual submitting the report; there may be confusion over what incidents should be reported; uncertainty may exist about the significance of certain events; and concern over the repercussions of reporting an incident both in terms of litigation and job security (Garrouste-Orgeas *et al.* 2012). Any of these uncertainties in the minds of potential reporters can lead to bias as to the type and number of incidents reported, that is, the data may not reflect the real world. To overcome these shortcoming, it is vital that reporters are given information and guidance about the types of incidents that should be reported and assurances regarding the confidentiality of the reports. However, it is also important that the report forms, be they paper or electronic, are made widely available, easy to complete and rapidly submitted.

Who should submit a report?

There are many sides to every story and narratives can be told from any number of different perspectives. Each narrative can be biased by the method used to report the incident as well as by the individual making the report. Often in team situations a single report can be made following a debriefing where all involved have been given the opportunity to speak and make their observations and thoughts known. However, these situations can be dominated by a single person or a small subgroup of individuals who can bias the report and leave vital viewpoints untold. Consequently, the clearest picture of any incident will come from multiple reports generated from differing standpoints; for this reason any person directly involved in or observing an error should be encouraged to report his or her observations.

What incidents should be reported?

It is our opinion that all incidents should be reported regardless of whether they are no-harm incidents (near misses) or cause patient harm (adverse incidents). Although some incidents may appear to be insignificant because they seem to be mundane, commonplace occurrences, or they do not cause harm, they can be critical in terms of highlighting larger problems within the system (Tripp 1993). All incidents that could have caused patient harm, including near misses, harmless hits, or harmful incidents, should be reported if a caregiver wants to achieve a full understanding of the system within which he or she works and prevent errors. For example, forgetting to open the pop-off valve on the breathing circuit of an anesthesia machine after manually sighing a patient, may not seem to be worthy of a report, especially if it does not harm the patient. After all, these incidents happen all the time, right? But if incidents such as this are not reported then we truly do not know how prevalent this or other patient safety incidents are in our work environment nor do we understand the circumstances that enable them.

Timing of reports: when should they be submitted?

When should reports be submitted? When harm has occurred to a patient or a caregiver the response, including the report, must be made immediately and should follow the guidelines for both care of the individual harmed and collection of information as outlined in Table 3.4. On the other hand, when situations or circumstances are identified that may cause patient harm, they too must be reported immediately and made broadly known throughout the workplace. Near misses, on the other hand, need not be reported immediately, but their occurrence and the circumstances under which they occurred must be documented and reported within a reasonable period of time. One possible approach for near misses is to post their occurrence at the end of a work day and then tabulate and summarize all such incidents at the end of the work week. An essential element is that these incidents be publicly reported soon after they occur. If too much time elapses between the occurrence of the incident and reporting it, then the facts and details of the incident may become blurred or lost or, worse yet, the incident is never reported and the opportunity to learn about the work environment is lost.

Capturing reports

Historically, voluntary reports have been handwritten descriptions of events that have been kept "in house" to help guide internal practices. This is clearly where the impact can be the greatest as the reports will have the most relevance and value. However, although some errors will be confined to and defined by the local environment and practices, many more will be generic, caused by universal human factors. This means that there is a need to track and analyze incidents both locally and globally to give a complete perspective and to maximize the collective learning potential. Collection of reports in this way leads to the formation of "big-data" sets and is greatly facilitated by the internet and smartphone technology. These technologies allow both rapid access to a reporting system and instant uploading of data. As a result, in human medicine at least, there is a move towards electronic capture, collation, and dissemination of incident reports producing large-scale regional or national databases. This approach is yet to be mirrored in veterinary medicine; however, there are several systems in use in other industries, including human anesthesia, that warrant discussion.

Table 3.4 An algorithm outlining the actions to take when an adverse incident has occurred.

Initial response	Analyze the event for pertinent domains and factors that must be considered when dealing with an incident (see Figure 3.4)
• Protect and manage the patient	
• Secure the records	
• Report the incident	• Perform root cause analysis
Gather information	• Identify contributing factors
• Assemble all of whom were involved in the incident	• Consider both human and latent factors
• Facilitate the interview process	• Determine accountability (see Figure 3.5)
Document the event	• Does the incident meet criteria for reporting?
• Identify pertinent features of the incident using tools such as the Ishikawa or fishbone diagram, that help to identify those general domains and contributing factors that must be considered when analyzing an adverse incident (see Figure 3.4)	Implement change
	• Implement corrective actions
	• Follow-up and monitor change
• Consider the possibility that substantial risk of harm may be persisting within the institution and determine how to prevent such risk	
• Review policies and guidelines relevant to the incident	

Adapted from: Kruskal, J.B., *et al.* (2008) Managing an acute adverse event in a radiology department. *Radiographics* 28: 1237–1250. With permission of the publisher.

Safety incident reporting in aviation

The Aviational Safety Reporting System (ASRS) is probably the most heralded current reporting system due to its scope and impact, so it warrants discussion. This longstanding system is operated by the National Aeronautics and Space Administration (NASA), with funding from the Federal Aviation Administration (FAA), and was developed to identify deficiencies and discrepancies in the US aerospace system. The initiating factor for its development was the high-profile incident on December 1, 1974, involving Trans World Airlines Flight 514, which crashed into a mountain as it descended towards Dulles Airport in Washington, DC, killing all 85 passengers and the seven crew members. Unfortunately, 6 weeks earlier a United Airlines flight had narrowly escaped the same fate, but this information was only disseminated within the United Airlines organization. This disaster tragically highlighted the need for an industry-wide method for collecting and disseminating database information regarding safety incidents; subsequently in 1976 the ASRS was established.

The aim of the Aviational Safety Reporting System is to collect, analyze and respond to safety reports submitted voluntarily by aviation workers, including personnel at all levels ranging from pilots to ground staff and flight attendants, air traffic controllers, mechanics, and management. All staff are actively encouraged to submit reports of any incident that they observe or are involved in that they believe compromises aviation safety. In addition to being voluntary the reports are guaranteed to be confidential, and non-punitive. The acceptance of this reporting system into aviation has been remarkable. At its inception it averaged almost 400 reports per month but has grown rapidly so that now it deals with over a million aviation safety incident reports a year, almost 6,000 reports per month (perhaps a slightly scary statistic if you're a frequent flyer!).

On an Aviational Safety Reporting System form the person reporting an incident is simply asked to describe the event or situation while "keeping in mind the topics shown below, discuss those which you feel are relevant and anything else you think is important." They are also asked to "include what you believe really caused the problem, and what can be done to prevent a recurrence, or correct the situation." The topics to be considered are "chain of events" (includes how the problem arose, how it was discovered, contributing factors, and corrective actions) and "human performance considerations" (includes perceptions, judgments, decisions, action or inaction, and any factors affecting the quality of human performance). This system of narrative reporting is in keeping with that used in the critical incident technique and attempts not to lead the person making the report into attributing the incident to any particular factor(s) and thus inadvertently biasing the report. Other pertinent details such as information about the reporter (their rank and duty, flying time, any certificates or ratings), the salient conditions and weather elements, light and visibility, location and their potential for collision are also collected in a separate section.

The Aviational Safety Reporting System has been extremely successful in maintaining aviation safety, an achievement that is supported by the fact that even though the number of passengers flying commercially was, by 2007, almost four times what it was in 1975, the fatality rate had declined by 96%, from an average annual absolute number of passenger fatalities of 166 in the mid-1970s to 39 in the decade from 2001 to 2010 (Savage 2013). The risk of a fatal accident has declined by 90% from about 0.8 per million departures in the mid-1970s to less than 0.1 today (Savage 2013). (Frequent flyers can breathe a sigh of relief!)

But the success of the Aviational Safety Reporting System is not attributable merely to the reporting system itself, but also to the manner in which the information is processed and the number of initiatives generated. Following a submission, the report is assigned to and rapidly screened by two specialist analysts. The incident described is categorized and the speed with which it will be processed is determined. The initial categorization allows multiple reports on the same event to be amalgamated into a single "record" in the database. Records that require further processing and analysis are identified and then coded using a specific taxonomy. If required, analysts are able to contact the reporter for further clarification of the submitted information; although confidential, the reports are not anonymous. After analysis a proof of submittal, in the form of a confirmation receipt, is sent to the reporter. At this point all identifying data are removed to ensure confidentiality and the anonymous reports are added to the open and freely accessible online database (see http://asrs.arc. nasa.gov/search/database.html).

The information received through the reports is disseminated throughout the aviation industry via a number of methods. Acutely hazardous situations are rapidly identified by analysts who are able to generate and issue "Alert Messages" for relaying safety information to the appropriate Federal Aviation Administration office or aviation authority so that evaluation and corrective actions can be taken. Time-critical safety information always triggers an immediate "Alert Bulletin," which is issued to all individuals who are in a position of authority and able to take action on the information; less urgent information is disseminated via "For Your Information"

notices. Where in-depth discussion of the safety information is required, teleconferences and other forums are used. Finally, the Aviational Safety Reporting System produces a number of publications and has been involved in a number of research studies regarding human factors in aviation. The monthly safety newsletter, CALLBACK (http://asrs.arc.nasa.gov/publications/callback.html), attempts to present significant safety information in an engaging and informal "lessons learned" fashion. This newsletter has almost 25,000 email subscribers and the various editions published in 2012 were downloaded over 300,000 times.

What about incident reporting in healthcare and anesthesia?

Australian Incident Monitoring System (AIMS)

The most longstanding incident reporting system in anesthesia is the Australian Incident Monitoring System (AIMS) coordinated by the Australian Patient Safety Foundation. Introduced in 1996 and using a single standard form, this monitoring system provides a means for reporting any incident or accident (actual or potential) in healthcare. Using a computer-based system, incidents are then classified using two unique classification systems developed by the Australian Patient Safety Foundation.

The Australian Incident Monitoring System arose from an incident monitoring study in anesthesia (AIMS-Anaesthesia) that began in 1988 (Runciman *et al.* 1993a, 1993b). Participating anesthetists were invited to anonymously and voluntarily report incidents using a specific form. In 1993, an issue of the journal *Anaesthesia and Intensive Care* published 30 papers relating to the first 2000 reports. These were the first large-scale papers to retrospectively analyze errors in anesthesia. Over the following seven years the AIMS-Anaesthesia project collated over 8000 reports. Since then the system has been broadened into an incident monitoring model that could be used on an institutional basis for all specialties. Since 1996 AIMS has been implemented in several Australian states and in individual health units. Over 200 healthcare organizations now voluntarily send reports to the Australian Incident Monitoring System.

As well as providing space for a narrative description of events the forms gather very detailed information from the reporter regarding generic types of incidents, contributing factors, outcomes, actions, and consequences via selecting options from predefined fields. The forms offer a highly sophisticated customizable data entry format that guides users through a cascade of natural questions and response choices that are structured and consistent. This level of highly structured reporting greatly facilitates large-scale data input to databases that are immediately ready for analysis. The data produced by these reports are designed to be analyzed using a specifically designed model, the Generic Reference Model (Runciman *et al.* 2006), which is based on Reason's model of complex system failure (Reason 1990). One criticism of this system is that the structured questions could influence the reports and thus introduce bias.

Other relevant reporting systems in healthcare

The United States does not have a national governmental reporting system, but almost half of the 50 state governments operate some form of incident reporting system. In addition there are a number of private and non-governmental initiatives via which multiple types of patient safety incidents can be reported. The most significant of these is the Sentinel Event Reporting System developed by the Joint Commission on Accreditation of Healthcare Organizations (JCAHO). Reports of incidents occurring in participating organizations are submitted to that organization via an online reporting tool in a manner similar to the Australian Incident Monitoring System. Other notable systems are the Institute for Safe Medication Practices (http://ismp. org/) and the United States Pharmacopeias Medication Error Reporting Program (MedMARx; https://www. medmarx.com), two programs for reporting medication-related incidents. Their successes are attributed to three factors that have been mentioned previously (Leape 2002): (1) those submitting reports are immune from disciplinary action if they report promptly; (2) the reports are not viewed as onerous; and (3) timely feedback of useful information is provided from expert analysis.

In the UK, prior to 2010, the National Patient Safety Agency (NPSA) developed the National Reporting and Learning System for collecting reports of safety incidents from all areas of care within the National Health Service (NHS). Because of changes within the National Health Service and reviews of the original reporting system, this system was replaced in March 2015 by the Serious Incident Framework for undertaking systems-based investigations that explore the problem (what?), the contributing factors to such problems (how?), and the root cause(s) or fundamental issues (why?) (NHS England Patient Safety Domain 2015). The system endorses and uses root cause analysis as a basis for investigations. The system's electronic form consists of categories with multiple questions with coded options defining where, when, how, and what occurred during any incident. Brief sections for narratives are embedded throughout the form.

Many other systems have been developed throughout the world both by national governments and private institutes (including the Anesthesia Incident Reporting System already mentioned in this chapter). Each system offers a variation on the themes outlined above; however, no single system is likely to be able to completely define an incident.

Analyzing patient safety incidents

As discussed at the beginning of this chapter, reporting an error is of little use if it is not analyzed appropriately. Poor analysis is detrimental and leads to rash decision-making, superficial fixes ("sticking plaster" over a surface wound and not investigating the injuries beneath), and often creates unnecessary layers of bureaucracy. In fact, a poorly performed analysis often just shifts blame further up or down the managerial-staff ladder.

The goal of analysis is to look beyond the error itself to the contributing factors that came together to allow that error to occur. Analysis should aim to provide, as both Tripp (1993) and Vincent (2004) term it, "a window into the system." It is unlikely that the whole truth will be illuminated, but rather some small part, hopefully the part with the most relevance and resonance, will be illuminated so that flaws within the system can be identified and hopefully corrected. In essence, analysis sets out to take context-specific data about an incident and devolve them into a concept-based assessment of the system in which the incident occurred. The end point of any analysis should be identification of solutions to system flaws that can be introduced to reduce the likelihood of error occurring in the future.

There are many investigative techniques that can be used for this purpose, each designed to "find" the underlying cause of an error. It is important to recognize that there is rarely a single causal factor or even a few causes responsible for any incident. In fact, analysis can often be a gross oversimplification as only a small number of causes will be identified even though there is a complex web of events and factors that interweave and combine to provide the circumstances specific to that incident. Dekker describes incident analysis as "constructing" and not "finding" contributing factors because "what we end up seeing as causal is a function of the questions we ask and the answers we set out to find" (Dekker 2011). Although this is a frustrating comment it is a cautionary one as it forces us to keep in mind that a single analytical method cannot lead to the whole truth of what happened in an incident. However, many methods can be used effectively to provide a "window" through which the system can be viewed and assessed.

Which incidents and errors should be analyzed?

Before we consider how to analyze incidents it is worth considering which incidents need to be investigated further. Clearly in an ideal world all errors would be investigated; however, analysis is a time-consuming business and analyzing all errors is not practicable.

All incidents that cause either significant patient harm or death clearly warrant analysis. What about lesser incidents, those that did not harm the patient? Some will be one-off events and some will be "repeat offenders." One method to help decide which incidents require more immediate investigation and analysis is the modified **Pareto chart**. This type of chart helps identify the incidents that occur most frequently and should be the focus of analysis.

To demonstrate this method we can examine incidents from a veterinary teaching hospital (Dr Daniel Fletcher, College of Veterinary Medicine, Cornell University, personal communication). In this study incidents were reported electronically over 6 months and subsequently analyzed. There were 95 incidents reported and grouped as follows (numbers in parentheses):

* Drug—wrong patient, drug, dose, route, or time (41).
* Communication—misidentified patient, confusion over orders or flow sheets, failure to share information (20).
* Oversights—judgment issues, missed diagnoses, misinterpretation of data, deviations from standard of care (10).
* System issues—delays, missed treatments, computer entry issue, protocol issue (9).

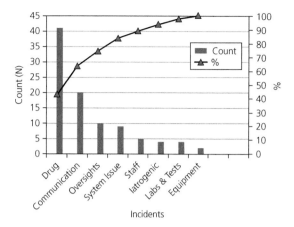

Figure 3.1 Modified Pareto chart showing categories of incidents recorded at a veterinary teaching hospital. According to the Pareto principle, the "Drug" category warrants further investigation as it accounts for 43% of all incidents, and the next most frequent error type is "Communication" at 20% of all incidents. The Pareto principle suggests that these two categories warrant deeper analysis.

* Staff—insufficient staff numbers, lack of access to needed staff, incident while training a staff member/clinician (5).
* Iatrogenic—a complication from a procedure or a treatment other than a drug (4).
* Labs and tests—lost specimens or documentation, mislabeled samples, results not reported, delays, improper studies (4).
* Equipment—inaccessibility, wrong equipment, failures, supply problems (2).

Figure 3.1 presents the data plotted in a modified Pareto chart. The left vertical axis is the count of each incident and is indicated by the height of the bars; the right vertical axis is the cumulative percentage of the total number of occurrences and is indicated by the line. The bars (items) are presented in descending order of frequency from left to right. These charts highlight the **Pareto principle**, which states that 20% of hazards cause 80% of incidents. The chart in Figure 3.1 indicates that the category with the most frequent incidents is "Drug" (i.e., medication error) as it accounts for 43% of all incidents, and the next most frequent error type is "Communication" at 20% of all incidents. The Pareto principle suggests that these two categories warrant deeper analysis, but how might we do this analysis?

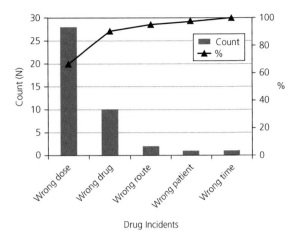

Drug Incidents

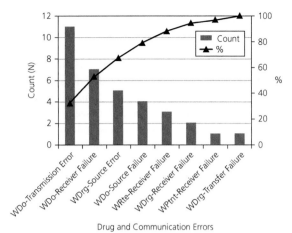

Drug and Communication Errors

Figure 3.2 A modified Pareto chart showing further analysis of the "Drug" category—drug errors—by sorting the data by wrong patient, wrong drug, wrong dose, wrong route, and wrong time. The chart graphically shows that the "wrong dose" category needs further analysis as it accounts for a little over 60% of the incidents.

Figure 3.3 Modified Pareto chart showing the "Wrong dose" data from Figure 3.2 and interaction with communication failures. This Pareto chart shows that the interaction of wrong dose with communication transmission error (information misunderstood or transmitted poorly, e.g., illegible handwriting) accounts for 32% of all incidents, and the combination of wrong dose plus transmission error plus receiver failure accounts for 52% of all errors and certainly warrants further examination as to their cause. Key: WDo = wrong dose; WDrg = wrong drug; WPtnt = wrong patient; WRte = wrong route.

If we focus only on the "Drug" category we can further categorize the errors into: wrong patient, wrong drug, wrong dose, wrong route, or wrong time. Categorizing the "Drug" data in this way yields the Pareto chart in Figure 3.2, which clearly shows that the "wrong dose" category accounts for 67% of all drug-related incidents.

This certainly helps shed light on this problem, but can we break it down further to get closer to the root causes of this problem? If we consider that medication errors are most often due to communication failures, such as discussed in Chapter 2 under "Communication: what it is and how it fails," we gain a deeper understanding of what may be the root causes of these medication incidents. Figure 3.3 presents data that show the interaction of wrong dose with communication transmission failure (information misunderstood or transmitted poorly, e.g., illegible handwriting). Transmission failures regarding the dose of a drug accounted for 32% of the incidents, and receiver failure regarding dose accounted for 20%. This gives a better idea of what causative factors should be explored further. However, we should recognize an unfortunate reality of this type of data and its analysis. At each step of the analysis process the number of incidents available for analysis decreased. The initial data set consisted of 95 incidents of which 42 were

categorized as "Drug." Further analysis of the drug data by communication failure yielded a total of 34 incidents. This decrease in numbers is due to the fact that some incident reports were incomplete, or it was difficult to assign some incidents to a particular category. Whatever the reason, the key message is that for incident reports to be useful they must be complete and have sufficient numbers for meaningful analysis. Nonetheless, modified Pareto charts offer a useful method in which data on harmless hits and near misses can be sorted in order of priority of analysis.

Analytical frameworks

Incidents are best analyzed within specific analytical frameworks. Analytical frameworks are scientific methods performed to uncover truths/realities or existing factors that promote or detract from the effective performance of a task. All such analyses should follow the basic five-step model of: (1) define the problem; (2) analyze cause and effect relationships; (3) identify solutions; (4) implement the best solutions; and (5) study the results.

Human factors and systems approach

Most authorities on error and patient safety recognize the importance of using a systems and human factors approach to error analysis. As a quick aside, the term "human factors" can be misleading as it suggests individuals are the focus of error analysis; although people may be observed or studied, the goal is to understand their cognitive and physical needs, and design systems and tools to better support their work tasks (Russ *et al.* 2013). This approach focuses on the entire system within which the error occurred.

The first question to answer is, what occurred and when? A sequence of events should be developed that identifies all of the decisions made and actions taken and how these changed the conditions in which the error took place. Special attention should be given to how the situation differed from what should have occurred or what was expected to occur, and what caused this change. Remember, when evaluating decision-making it is all too easy to unfairly criticize it using the "retrospectoscope" (hindsight bias).

Subsequent analysis should aim to answer the following questions:

- What were the goals, focuses of attention, and knowledge of the people involved at the time?
- Did any of these collide or conflict?
- How was the situation interpreted by those involved?
- What influenced their decision-making and actions?

It is important both to highlight the differences between what occurred and what should have occurred, and to define possible links and similarities between apparently disparate incidents. This helps to highlight specific weaknesses within a system that descriptions of differing incidents might not immediately highlight. Only by doing this can an appropriate solution or solutions be developed.

Root cause analysis (RCA)

Just after the birth of the critical incident technique the process of root cause analysis (RCA) was conceived. Root cause analysis was developed initially as a problem-solving tool for engineers in industry. Like the critical incident technique the principle is to identify those underlying factors (or root causes) that enabled a problem to occur thus enabling implementation of corrective measures. The invention of root cause analysis is credited to Sakichi Toyoda, a Japanese inventor and industrialist, and founder of Toyota Industries Corporation. His original brainstorming technique, first used in Toyota's manufacturing processes in 1958, was simply to "ask why five times." This approach asks again and again why a problem occurred, and does so systematically using the answer from the previous question to form the next question until the root cause of the problem is identified. Generally about five "whys" are required to get a good idea about the underlying cause. The following are examples of how a root cause analysis of an anesthetic incident could be conducted.

Incident 1: The patient regained consciousness during surgery

Why? The vaporizer was not adequately filled.

Why? The anesthetic machine had not been checked prior to anesthesia.

Why? The anesthetist did not have time to check the machine.

Why? The anesthetist was scheduled to do too many cases.

Why? The anesthesia service was short staffed.

This process produces a linear set of causal relationships that can be used to create solutions to the problem being analyzed. Of course this is a massive oversimplification as often the causes of error are multifactorial, and thus have many root causes. In fact the question pathway could follow many different courses, each giving a completely different set of answers that could be equally valid.

Incident 2: The patient regained consciousness during surgery

Why? The anesthetist did not notice that the patient had become light.

Why? The anesthetist was distracted.

Why? The anesthetist was fatigued and was trying to teach a student at the same time.

Why? The anesthetist had been on call the night before and had not been given a chance to recuperate.

Why? Being on call and then working a day shift is expected behavior in veterinary medicine.

It is also important to recognize that this can sometimes be an endless exercise because no matter how deep you go there is always at least one more root cause you can look for. At some point a judgment has to be made that the "root cause" is the last meaningful, fundamental cause, one to which there is an effective solution or solutions to the problem. Once that cause is removed or corrected, and the incident does not recur, then a simple actionable level has been reached where interventions or changes to the system can be made.

Incident 3: The patient regained consciousness during surgery

Why? The anesthetist did not have any injectable anesthetic agent ready when the patient moved.

Why? Additional injectable anesthetic is not on the pre-anaesthetic equipment list.

At this point there is a simple solution, that of changing the set-up list to ensure all anesthetic protocols include an additional amount of injectable anesthetic agent.

This is still an oversimplification of the problem as each of the answers to each of the whys could also have a number of causes. Therefore the person or persons doing the analysis should return to each answer at each level and ask why again and again until the possible causes are identified.

To get a good idea of all the underlying root causes a thorough approach is needed, one that involves a good working knowledge of the process and the system involved as well as the incident itself. To deal with this complexity root cause analysis has evolved considerably over time and a number of methods and tools have been developed to assist analysis (Diller *et al.* 2014; Kruskal *et al.* 2008; Wald & Shojania 2001). This has made it possible to use this analytical method in a variety of different circumstances. One of the most popular types of tools are diagrams that help break down the process and its analysis into component parts.

Causal tree

The causal tree is a diagram with the incident at the top of the tree. All possible answers as to why the incident occurred are written below. Why is then asked for each of these questions and all possible answers are written in. This is performed until each branch of the tree has reached a simple actionable level or the last meaningful answer, and the potential causes at each level of the tree have been exhaustively identified.

Mind map

This is a diagram much like a causal tree, and is meant to visually organize information by representing relationships between a problem and its root causes. The incident is placed in the center and major contributing factors or ideas branch outwards with other contributing factors or ideas branching off from the main branches. Its structure is such that it does not assign levels of importance to the contributing factors or ideas.

Reality charting

Reality charting is a proprietary (Gano 2008) method that is meant to achieve greater insight to the "reality" of an event or process by requiring that for each "why" question there is at least one action and one condition. Actions are causes that interact with conditions to cause an effect. Conditions are causes that exist in time prior to an action; both actions and conditions come together to cause an effect. This method displays all known causes from the perspective of all participants involved in an incident, and helps to identify interplay and relationships between the causes. It is a method that recognizes that people can view the exact same incident and yet see very different causes (Gano 2002).

Ishikawa diagram or fishbone diagram

The Ishikawa diagram is one of seven tools of quality management. It was developed by Kaoru Ishikawa, who was influenced by a series of lectures given by W. Edwards Deming to Japanese engineers and scientists in 1950, and who pioneered quality management processes in the Kawasaki shipyards in the 1960s. The other six tools of quality management are: check sheet, control chart, histogram, Pareto chart, scatter diagram, and stratification (flow chart or run chart).

In the fishbone diagram the "head" of the fish represents the incident while branching off the "backbone" are the "ribs" representing domains of contributing factors (Figure 3.4). The domains are traditionally grouped as methods, materials, equipment, manpower, and environment, but other categories can be used depending on the nature of the organization. The fishbone diagram in Figure 3.4 uses the domains involved in error incidents as identified by Reason and Diller and also used in Figure 2.1. Factors implicated in the incident are then added within their corresponding domains. This type of diagram is widely used in incident analysis, but it must be kept in mind that it may not demonstrate all of the causal relationships between domains of contributing factors and root causes. This is not because of a shortcoming of this tool, but more a function of the "questions we ask and the answers we set out to find" (Dekker 2011).

Systems walk

A timeline is created to depict the step-by-step sequence of different elements in a system's process. This approach is often used to identify unnecessary, redundant, or

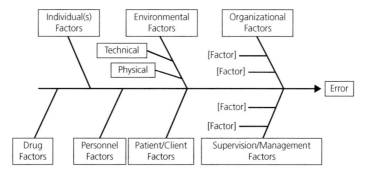

Figure 3.4 Fishbone or Ishikawa diagram (also known as a cause-and-effect diagram) is a tool for identifying the various domains and contributing factors involved in an incident. The "head" of the diagram is the error, whatever it may be. The ribs are the domains as identified by Reason and Diller, and as used in Figure 2.1. Factors within each domain that contributed to the error are identified through processes of brainstorming and root cause analysis.

failing steps in a process. For a discussion of how this process might be used in veterinary anesthesia see "Evaluating the process of anesthesia: systems walk" in Chapter 8.

What method might be best for veterinary anesthesia?

There is no gold standard method for reporting and analyzing critical incidents in medicine or industry let alone veterinary anesthesia. All of the previously mentioned methods could be successfully integrated into larger veterinary organizations given time and resources, but they may not be ideal for smaller practices. Probably the key is not what method is used (all methods can be performed either well or badly), but to properly apply whatever method is used while taking into account the system being analyzed and the human factors that are involved. The domains and factors identified in Figures 2.1 and 3.4 can serve as templates for analysis.

We believe that all incidents should be reported even though some may not be particularly dramatic or obvious—seemingly only straightforward accounts of very commonplace events that occur daily in anesthesia. For example, after giving a patient a sigh and then failing to open the pop-off valve on the breathing circuit is an incident that has the potential to cause serious harm to a patient. Bringing the wrong patient to the anesthesia induction area because of confusion about the owner's last name or the patient's breed, is a potentially serious incident, even if the error is caught before the patient is sedated or anesthetized. Drawing up the wrong drug for a patient has the potential to cause harm and must be reported. Again, these types of

incidents, of which there are many and that vary depending on the practice, must be made known if a practice is to develop a patient safety culture; all of these errors may be indicative of system-wide shortcomings that are prone to error generation (Tripp 1993). The reports should contain a detailed description of what occurred and how the events or actions deviated significantly, either positively or negatively, from normal or expected practice (Edvardsson 1992). Analysis of incident reports requires clinical expertise and a solid understanding of the task, the context, and the many factors that may influence and contribute to an incident.

Analysis of the person(s) at the sharp end: accountability

When adverse incidents occur they evoke a variety of intense emotions including embarrassment, fear of repercussions, guilt, and a tendency by many to seek out and "blame and shame" the person(s) who committed the error. When such incidents occur and emotions run high, how can we resolve the many issues that arise and need resolution? Is there a process we can use in the heat of the moment that assures important issues and considerations are not overlooked so that the incident is not made worse because of a failure to take the right steps at the right time? Such guidelines do exist and have been used in human medicine. Table 3.4 describes one such approach that we believe is as applicable to veterinary medicine as it is to human medicine (Kruskal *et al.* 2008).

As previously stated, people do not go to work with the intention of making errors or causing harm. But we

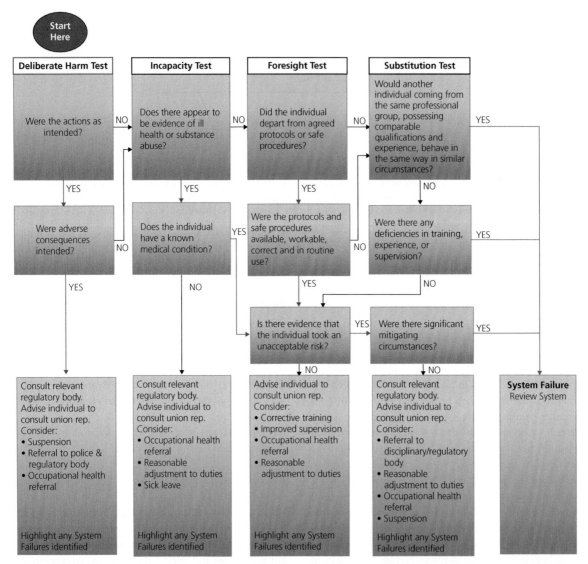

Figure 3.5 An Incident Decision Tree is used to determine accountability of the individual or individuals involved in an incident. It is worked through separately for each individual involved and starts at the Deliberate Harm Test. The Tree is easy to follow with the YES/NO responses guiding the analysis. Each test requires that any system failures that are identified must be highlighted. If an individual "passes" all of the tests, then the error is judged to be a system failure and attention must then focus on the system. From: Meadows, S., Baker, K., & Butler, J. (2005) The Incident Decision Tree: Guidelines for action following patient safety incidents. In: Henriksen, K., et al. (eds) *Advances in Patient Safety: From Research to Implementation. Volume 4: Programs, Tools, and Products*. Rockville, MD: Agency for Healthcare Research and Quality, pp. 387–399. Used with permission from Agency for Healthcare Research and Quality and the UK National Health Service.

must recognize that it is the individual(s) dealing directly with the patient who causes the error. Again, malicious intent and wrongdoing are never to be condoned, but what process can we use that is just and fair for determining accountability and identifies the steps

that should be taken regarding the caregiver who erred? The Incident Decision Tree (Figure 3.5) graphically identifies steps that must be taken to determine if the caregiver intended deliberate harm, took unnecessary risks with patient management, or was in any way incapacitated and thus unable to properly perform the task. The Decision Tree guides the analytical process beyond the issues of willful intent to cause harm and impairment and thus helps to guide us to the most appropriate course of action when in the heat of the moment we have to make important personnel decisions.

Conclusion

Some incidents may not be dramatic or obvious; they may seem to be nothing more than straightforward accounts of very commonplace events that occur in the daily practice of veterinary anesthesia. But they can be critical indicators of underlying trends, motives, and structures within a veterinary practice, factors that can and do lead to errors. These incidents should be reported, analyzed, and the information learned should be shared throughout the veterinary community so that there can be accelerated moments of learning and growth of self-awareness, seminal moments in the process of change (Cope & Watts 2000).

References

Baker, G.R., *et al.* (2004) The Canadian adverse events study: The incidence of adverse events among hospital patients in Canada. *Canadian Medical Association Journal* **170**(11): 1678–1686.

Betsch, C., *et al.* (2011) The influence of narrative v. statistical information on perceiving vaccination risks. *Medical Decision Making* **31**(5): 742–753.

Billings, C. (1998) *Incident Reporting Systems in Medicine and Experience With the Aviation Safety Reporting System*. Chicago, IL: National Patient Safety Foundation at the AMA.

Blum, L.L. (1971) Equipment design and "human" limitations. *Anesthesiology* **35**(1): 101–102.

Cook, R.I., Woods, W.D., & Miller, C. (1998) *A Tale of Two Stories: Contrasting Views of Patient Safety*. Chicago, IL: National Health Care Safety Council of the National Patient Safety Foundation at the AMA.

Cooper, J.B. (1996) Is voluntary reporting of critical events effective for quality assurance? *Anesthesiology* **85**(5): 961–964.

Cooper, J.B., *et al.* (1978) Preventable anesthesia mishaps: A study of human factors. *Anesthesiology* **49**(6): 399–406.

Cope, J. & Watts, G. (2000) Learning by doing – an exploration of experience, critical incidents and reflection in entrepreneurial learning. *International Journal of Entrepreneurial Behaviour & Research* **6**(3): 104–124.

Cullen, D.J., *et al.* (2000) Prevention of adverse drug events: A decade of progress in patient safety. *Journal of Clinical Anesthesia* **12**(8): 600–614.

Dahlstrom, M.F. (2014) Using narratives and storytelling to communicate science with nonexpert audiences. *Proceedings of the National Academy of Sciences of the United States of America* **111**(Suppl. 4): 13614–13620.

Dekker, S. (2011) *Patient Safety: A Human Factors Approach*. Boca Raton, FL: CRC Press, Taylor & Francis Group.

Diller, T., *et al.* (2014) The human factors analysis classification system (HFACS) applied to health care. *American Journal of Medical Quality* **29**(3): 181–190.

Dutton, R.P. (2014) Improving safety through incident reporting. *Current Anesthesiology Reports* **4**(2): 84–89.

Edvardsson, B. (1992) Service breakdowns: A study of critical incidents in an airline. *International Journal of Service Industry Management* **3**(4): 17–29.

Flanagan, J.C. (1954) The critical incident technique. *Psychological Bulletin* **51**(4): 327–358.

Gano, D.L. (2002) *Four steps to effective solutions*. Milwaukee: American Society for Quality, 97 pp.

Gano, D.L. (2008) *Apollo Root Cause Analysis – a New Way of Thinking*, 3rd edn. Richland, WA: Apollonian,.

Garrouste-Orgeas, M., *et al.* (2012) Overview of medical errors and adverse events. *Annals of Intensive Care* **2**: 2–10.

Gerrig, R.J. (1993) *Experiencing Narrative Worlds: On the Psychological Activities of Reading*. New Haven, CT: Yale University Press.

Hofmeister, E.H., *et al.* (2014) Development, implementation and impact of simple patient safety interventions in a university teaching hospital. *Veterinary Anaesthesia & Analgesia* **41**(3): 243–248.

Hogan, H., *et al.* (2012) Preventable deaths due to problems in care in English acute hospitals: A retrospective case record review study. *BMJ Quality & Safety* **21**(9): 737–745.

James, J.T. (2013) A new, evidence-based estimate of patient harms associated with hospital care. *Journal of Patient Safety* **9**(3): 122–128.

Kennerly, D.A., *et al.* (2014) Characterization of adverse events detected in a large health care delivery system using an enhanced global trigger tool over a five-year interval. *Health Services Research* **49**(5): 1407–1425.

Kruskal, J.B., *et al.* (2008) Managing an acute adverse event in a radiology department. *Radiographics* **28**(5): 1237–1250.

Leape, L.L. (2002) Reporting of adverse events. *New England Journal of Medicine* **347**(20): 1633–1638.

NHS England Patient Safety Domain (2015) *Serious incident framework – supporting learning to prevent recurrence*. London: National Health Service.

Reason, J.T. (1990) *Human Error*. Cambridge: Cambridge University Press.

Rochlin, G.I. (2012) Expert operators and critical tasks. In: *Trapped in the net: the unanticipated consequences of computerization*. Princeton, NJ: Princeton University Press, 126 pp.

Runciman, W.B., *et al.* (1993a) Crisis management—validation of an algorithm by analysis of 2000 incident reports. *Anaesthesia and Intensive Care* **21**(5): 579–592.

Runciman, W.B., *et al.* (1993b) The Australian incident monitoring study. system failure: An analysis of 2000 incident reports. *Anaesthesia and Intensive Care* **21**(5): 684–695.

Runciman, W.B., *et al.* (2006) An integrated framework for safety, quality and risk management: An information and incident management system based on a universal patient safety classification. *Quality & Safety in Health Care* **15**(Suppl. 1): i82–i90.

Russ, A.L., *et al.* (2013) The science of human factors: Separating fact from fiction. *BMJ Quality & Safety* **22**(10): 802–808.

Savage, I. (2013) Comparing the fatality risks in United States transportation across modes and over time. *Research in Transportation Economics* **43**(1): 9–22.

Stephens, G.J., *et al.* (2010) Speaker-listener neural coupling underlies successful communication. *Proceedings of the National Academy of Sciences of the United States of America* **107**(32): 14425–14430.

Tripp, D. (1993) *Critical Incidents in Teaching: Developing Professional Judgement*. London: Routledge.

Vincent, C.A. (2004) Analysis of clinical incidents: A window on the system not a search for root causes. *Quality & Safety in Health Care* **13**(4): 242–243.

Wald, H. & Shojania, K.G. (2001) Root cause analysis. In: *Making Health Care Safer: A Critical Analysis of Patient Safety Practices* (eds K.G. Shojania, B.W. Duncan, K.M. McDonald, & R.M. Wachter). Rockville, MD: Agency for Health Care Research and Quality, pp. 51–56.

Wells, C.G. (1986) *The Meaning Makers: Children Learning Language and using Language to Learn*, 1st edn. Portsmouth, NH: Heinemann.

Winterbottom, A., *et al.* (2008) Does narrative information bias individual's decision making? A systematic review. *Social Science & Medicine (1982)* **67**(12): 2079–2088.

CHAPTER 4

Equipment and Technical Errors in Veterinary Anesthesia

Knowledge rests not upon truth alone, but upon error also.
Carl Gustav Jung (1875–1961)

Equipment and our interactions with it play a central role in modern anesthetic practice. Anesthetic machines and vaporizers provide measured flows of anesthetic gases and vapors while airway equipment and breathing systems allow these gases to be transported to and from the patient. Ventilators support respiration whilst pumps and syringe drivers administer intravenous fluids and drugs. Electronic monitoring equipment gives measurements and readings that provide information on the patient's physiological function.

Equipment can be even more fundamental. For example, rarely do we think of catheters as equipment; more often they are thought of as supply items in part because they are disposable. Nonetheless, catheters used for intravascular cannulation are an important feature of anesthetic management and, although they have the potential for great good, they also have the potential to cause harm (Hofmeister *et al.* 2014; Singleton *et al.* 2005). Consequently, the proper use of catheters requires eye-hand coordination, knowledge of how the catheter is designed and meant to be used, and knowledge of the patient's anatomy. Knowledge of the hazards associated with intravascular catheters is gained through education and training, the same elements that make it possible for us to use other pieces of anesthetic equipment.

So the roles of equipment in anesthesia are legion, but as technology and technical skills have become more and more integrated into the process of anesthesia the potential for misuse, malfunction, and failure of each piece of equipment remains. But how often does equipment actually malfunction or fail? Before answering that question we should first try to define

what equipment failure is. This sounds like a simple task, but as Webb has stated:

> It is difficult to define "true" equipment failure as almost every aspect of equipment design, manufacture, supply, installation, maintenance, testing and use involves humans and thus anything which goes wrong has the potential to be due to a human error of some sort.
>
> *Webb et al. (1993).*

For the purposes of this chapter we have basically considered equipment error as errors that center around the use, misuse, or malfunction of a piece of equipment (anything that is not a person or patient).

Even when ignoring the lack of a clear-cut definition, the frequency with which equipment or technical error occurs in anesthetic practice is not clear even in human anesthesia; like many error-related issues it is underreported. In one retrospective study of 83,000 anesthetics performed over a period of 4 years (1996–2000) in a Norwegian hospital, the incidence of reported "equipment or technical" problems was 0.23% for general anesthetics and 0.05% for locoregional anesthetics (with a total of 157 problems being reported) (Fasting & Gisvold 2002). Most of these problems were considered "trivial," having little effect on the patients or their care, but almost 30% (45/157) caused some harm to patients, for example, a period of hypoxemia, hypercapnia, or hypoperfusion. None of the problems were considered to have caused lasting harm. About one-third (49/157) of the problems were associated with anesthetic machines, and in about one-quarter (40/157) of these events "human error" was considered a causal factor, and almost half of these events were associated with

Errors in Veterinary Anesthesia, First Edition. John W. Ludders and Matthew McMillan.
© 2017 John Wiley & Sons, Inc. Published 2017 by John Wiley & Sons, Inc.

anesthetists not adequately following pre-anesthetic checks (Fasting & Gisvold 2002).

Other studies have generally analyzed incident reports but could not give an estimate of incidence due to the lack of a denominator. Cooper used a modified critical incident technique (see "Critical incident technique (CIT)" in Chapter 3) to gather reports of human error and equipment "failure" from 139 anesthesia providers (anesthesiologists, residents, and nurse-anesthetists) (Cooper *et al.* 1984). Of the 1089 descriptions of "preventable incidents" that were collected, only 11% represented true equipment failure while another 13% involved disconnection of the patient from the breathing system or disconnection of the breathing system from the anesthetic machine. Table 4.1 shows the distribution of equipment failures based upon the type of equipment used. Interestingly, Cooper found that equipment failure was less likely to be involved in an adverse patient outcome than human error. This led to him to conclude "perhaps people have more difficulty detecting their own errors than failures of their equipment" (Cooper *et al.* 1984).

Webb *et al.* (1993) analyzed and reported on equipment failures identified in the first 2000 incident reports submitted to the Australian Incident Monitoring System (AIMS) (see Chapter 3). This yielded 177 incidents of equipment failure (just under 9% of the incidents reported). Problems associated with failure of unidirectional valves (46 in total), monitoring equipment (42), and ventilators (32) were the most commonly reported equipment failures. Of these 177 incidents 97 (55%) were considered to be potentially life threatening, with 62 detectable by standard anesthetic monitoring.

More recently Cassidy *et al.* (2011) reported on anesthetic equipment incidents reported to the UK National Health Service's National Reporting and Learning System between the years 1996 and 2000. Of the 195,812 incidents reported from the anesthetic and surgical specialties, 1029 incidents of anesthetic equipment failure were identified. Of these about 40% (410) were associated with monitoring equipment, 18% (185) with ventilators, 10% (99) with leaks, and 5% (53) associated with fluid pumps. The large majority of incidents (89%) did not cause patient harm, but 2.9% (30 incidents) led to moderate or severe harm. Most reports were associated with equipment faults or failure, but a small proportion were clearly or most likely the result of user error. Unfamiliarity with equipment, failure to follow checklists, and failure to act on reports of temperamental equipment were recurrently cited causal factors. It is worth noting that an additional 215 airway equipment reports were identified but not analyzed.

The most recent assessment of equipment failure in the United States was published by the American Society of Anesthesiologists' Closed Claim Project. Mehta *et al.* (2013) reviewed just over 6000 closed claim reports associated with anesthesia care that were filed between 1970 and 2011, and more specifically those reports associated with anesthesia gas delivery equipment. This subset of cases was analyzed further and classified as primarily due to: (1) equipment failure

Table 4.1 Distribution of equipment failures according to type of equipment involved.

	Number of incidents	Percentage of all equipment failures (rounded to whole numbers)
Breathing circuit	26	23
Monitoring device	22	19
Ventilator	17	15
Anesthesia machine	16	14
Airway device	14	12
Laryngoscope	11	10
Other	9	8
Total	115	

From: Cooper, J.B., et al. (1984) An analysis of major errors and equipment failures in anesthesia management: considerations for prevention and detection. *Anesthesiology* **60**(1): 34–42. Reprinted with permission of the publisher.

(unexpected failure despite routine maintenance and previous uneventful use); (2) provider error (faults associated with maintenance, preparation or deployment of a device); or (3) failure to follow appropriate pre-anesthesia check-out procedures (faults that would have been detected had procedures been adhered to). One hundred and fifteen claims were identified, with 80% of those occurring between 1990 and 2011, and involving vaporizers, supplemental oxygen delivery equipment, and breathing systems. True equipment failure occurred in only 5% of cases, of which one-third were considered preventable had pre-anesthesia checkouts been properly performed (Mehta *et al.* 2013).The remaining significant issues were attributed to provider error, including inadequate setting of alarms, improvised oxygen delivery systems, and misdiagnosis or mistreatment of breathing circuit events.

So what about in veterinary anesthesia? Unfortunately the picture is likely to be far worse. A number of factors are likely to increase the incidence of equipment and technical error in veterinary anesthesia, including much less education and training compared to human anesthesia, less stringent procedural guidelines (such as pre-anesthesia checks), lack of standardization for anesthesia equipment such as anesthesia machines, and lack of policies regarding maintenance and servicing of equipment. The one mitigating factor may be reduced complexity of equipment in the veterinary sector and potentially a lower reliance on technology, especially in the general practice arena.

What follows are some examples of equipment error in veterinary anesthesia.

Cases

Case 4.1

A 6-year-old gelding weighing 514 kg was brought to a referral center for laryngeal surgery to correct airway problems that were causing poor performance. On the day of surgery the horse's vital signs were: heart and respiratory rates 36 beats per minute and 16 breaths per minute, respectively; capillary refill time of less than 2 seconds; and moist and pink mucous membranes. Rectal temperature was 38 °C, hematocrit was 35%, and total protein was 62 g L^{-1}. Physical examination was unremarkable and all other blood work was within normal limits for the referral hospital's clinical laboratory.

While the horse was in its stall, the anesthetist inserted a catheter into its left jugular vein and secured it in position. Thirty minutes later the horse was walked to the anesthesia induction area where its mouth was rinsed with water to flush out food debris in preparation for orotracheal intubation. The horse was then injected with detomidine (3 mg) via the jugular vein catheter. As soon as the catheter was flushed with heparinized saline the horse stumbled, dropped to its knees, and then quickly stood and shook its head.

Thirteen minutes later, during which the horse seemed normal for a sedated horse, it was injected with diazepam (15 mg, intravenously) followed 8 minutes later by ketamine (1.2 g, intravenously). The induction was described as rough in that the horse fell suddenly and atypically to the floor. It was intubated (using a 30-mm internal diameter endotracheal tube) then hoisted by his legs onto the surgical table. The endotracheal tube was attached to a large animal anesthesia machine, and mechanical ventilation was initiated (7 breaths min^{-1}, tidal volume 7 L) delivering halothane (3%) in oxygen (7 L min^{-1}). At this time the anesthetist considered the possibility that the catheter was in the carotid artery and that all drugs had been inadvertently injected into it. As a consequence no additional injections were made through that catheter and another catheter was inserted into the right jugular vein through which all subsequent drugs and fluids were administered.

Throughout the course of anesthesia the horse's heart rate ranged between 32 and 35 beats per minute and mean arterial blood pressure ranged between 60 and 80 mmHg. Results of arterial blood gas analysis at 30 and 60 minutes after induction were acceptable for an anesthetized horse in lateral recumbency. Sixty-seven minutes after induction, an infusion of dobutamine was started to treat arterial hypotension (mean arterial blood pressure 65 mmHg). After 95 minutes of anesthesia, all monitoring devices were disconnected from the horse and he was turned from lateral recumbency to dorsal recumbency for the last stage of the surgical procedure. During repositioning the horse was administered ketamine to maintain anesthesia (two 200-mg boluses). Thirty minutes after being positioned in dorsal recumbency the horse was extubated for 10 minutes so as to facilitate surgical exploration of the larynx. During this time anesthesia was again augmented with ketamine (one 400-mg bolus), and ventilation was assisted intermittently as the surgical procedure allowed. At the end of surgery the horse was moved to a recovery stall where positive pressure ventilation was continued with a Hudson demand valve until the horse started breathing spontaneously.

By 30 minutes after discontinuing anesthesia the horse started to breathe spontaneously, but recovery seemed slow for the type of anesthesia and surgery. After 70 minutes in the recovery stall the horse started to show signs of seizure activity with extensor rigidity. The horse was re-intubated and positive pressure ventilation was commenced with the Hudson demand valve. Although arterial blood gas analysis indicated normocarbemia ($P_a CO_2$ 44 mmHg), the horse was hypoxemic ($P_a O_2$ 47 mmHg). Diazepam was administered to control seizure activity, but its effect lasted only 10 to 20 minutes. It was decided to induce anesthesia using thiamylal (2 g) in glycerol guaifenesin (GG; 5% solution) administered to effect to stop seizure activity, and then maintain anesthesia and control seizure activity with pentobarbital (3.8 g, intravenously). Furosemide was administered to reduce cerebral edema, and dimethyl sulfoxide (DMSO) was given for its anti-inflammatory and oxygen radical scavenging effects. Despite these efforts the horse's condition deteriorated over time. After 13 hours in the recovery stall the horse was euthanized at the owner's request.

At necropsy a 2 × 2 cm area of yellow discoloration on the surface of the left occipital cortex was found as well as diffuse vascular congestion of the left cerebral hemisphere. A cross-section of the brain revealed bilateral yellow discoloration and malacia of the entire hippocampus and yellow discoloration of the deeper aspects of the left occipital cortex in the region supplied by the caudal cerebral artery (Figure 4.1).

Initial analysis of the case

Upon initial analysis this case seemed to be primarily an example of a skill-based error in that the act of catheterizing a horse relates to technical performance and proper execution of the task. Such errors suggest inadequate training and experience in performing this type of procedure. However, focusing only on the anesthetist ignores other factors that may have contributed to this error and warrant deeper investigation. Indeed, subsequent assessment of this case revealed that the horse was catheterized under conditions that would have made this task challenging for anyone regardless of training and experience.

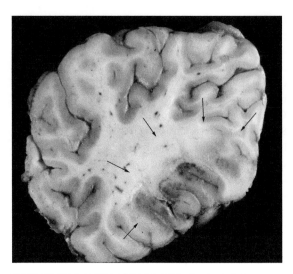

Figure 4.1 Cross-section of the horse's brain at necropsy showing injury to the left occipital lobe after accidental injection into the left carotid artery of detomidine as a premedicant and ketamine plus diazepam for induction of anesthesia. Black arrows indicate the boundaries of the lesion consisting of discoloration and malacia of the entire hippocampus and discoloration of the deeper aspects of the left occipital cortex.

The stall was dimly lit, which made it difficult for the anesthetist to see the jugular vein and the color of blood flowing out of the catheter. The anesthetist, in trying to comply with the surgeon's request that catheters be inserted into the jugular vein as far from the surgical site as possible, inserted it close to the thoracic inlet, a location that imposed some anatomic constraints on catheterization. Inserting the catheter with its tip directed cranially also made it difficult to distinguish venous blood flow from arterial blood flow. These latter two factors posed two challenges for the anesthetist: the hand holding the catheter was forced by the point of the horse's shoulder to direct the catheter at an angle that made it more likely it would be inserted through the jugular vein and into the carotid artery. Furthermore, inserting the catheter parallel to and in the direction of carotid arterial blood flow increased the likelihood that arterial blood would not pulse out of the catheter thus making it appear more like venous blood flow and giving a false sense of having inserted the catheter into the jugular vein.

This case is also an example of a rule-based error in that there was misapplication of a rule that went something like: "*when anesthetizing a horse for surgery of the larynx, insert the catheter at a location on the jugular vein that is far from the surgical site.*" But there was no matching of the conditional prerequisite—**if**—with the action portion—**then**—of the rule that goes something like: "**if** a drug is injected into a horse's jugular vein and the horse immediately shows central nervous system (CNS) signs, e.g., stumbles or collapses, **then** one must suspect the injection was into the carotid artery and not the jugular vein." This latter rule, had it even been made explicit in the first place and properly followed, would have forced the operator to check the location of the catheter. Eventually this check did happen, but only after the induction drugs had been injected through the catheter and caused a very rough, atypical induction. All of this suggests that the anesthetist was solely responsible for this error, but as usual there are other factors to consider.

Investigation of the case

For this particular type of laryngeal surgery the surgeons had a standing order that all catheters inserted into the jugular vein were to be inserted as far distally as possible on the horse's neck so as not to interfere with the surgical site; this was a departure from the standard catheterization practice that was in effect at this equine hospital. The usual practice was to shave hair from the junction of the upper and middle thirds of the cervical jugular vein, wash the area until clean, and then insert the catheter with its tip directed toward the heart (Box 4.1).

At first glance this standing order seems quite reasonable. However, it posed hazards that came to the fore when an individual who lacked the requisite skills and experience performed the catheterization and did so under challenging environmental (poor lighting) and physical conditions (hand position and equine anatomy). The primary hazard was unintentional catheterization of the carotid artery because in the caudal third of the equine neck the carotid artery is close to the jugular vein and the omohyoid muscle does not separate the two vessels at this level as it does starting about midway up the neck. The omohyoid muscle somewhat serves as an anatomic barrier and lessens—but does not eliminate—the likelihood of inserting a catheter into the carotid artery.

Any number of adverse effects may occur following intracarotid injection of drugs, including vasoconstriction, thrombosis, intravascular crystallization of injected

---

Box 4.1 Thoughts on variations in catheterization practice.

One of the delights in writing this book has been our cross-ocean collaboration and the insights we have gained concerning differences in anesthetic management. Jugular catheterization in the horse is one example. In the UK a common practice is to insert the catheter with its tip directed upstream, toward the head. In the United States the common practice is to direct the tip toward the heart. Justifications have been presented for both approaches.

Directing the catheter tip toward the head rather than the heart reduces the risk that if the injection cap comes off the catheter during induction, air will be entrained into the catheter and create a fatal air embolus. The other approach, that of directing the catheter tip toward the heart, usually makes it quickly obvious that the carotid artery, and not the jugular vein, has been catheterized; inserting the catheter toward the head makes it difficult to distinguish carotid arterial blood flow from venous blood flow because the pulsatile nature of arterial blood flow from the carotid is dampened out.

Both approaches have merit. Indeed, one of us has witnessed the death of a horse due to an air embolus when the injection cap came off the hub of the catheter that was directed toward the heart. We have also seen catheters inserted into the carotid when the intent was to insert them into the jugular vein, and there was no pulsing of blood to indicate that such was the case. Unfortunately, adverse incidents can occur as a result of these catheter errors.

---

compounds, endothelial inflammation, and direct cytotoxicity (Valentine *et al.* 2009). Intracarotid injections of alpha-2 agonists, such as xylazine or detomidine, have near-immediate adverse central nervous system effects, possibly due to drug-induced cerebral vasoconstriction. When alpha-2 agonists are injected into the carotid artery, horses usually immediately show signs, such as stumbling and falling to their knees, as did the horse in this case; horses may fall into lateral recumbency and remain recumbent and unresponsive for several minutes. Most horses seem to recover without long-lasting effects. In the patient of this case the subsequent injection of ketamine into the carotid artery for induction of anesthesia may have been the additional factor needed to produce significant injury to the left occipital lobe of the brain. Ketamine is both hyperosmolar and acidic, but it also has a direct cytotoxic effect that may be due to the drug itself or the preservative benzethonium (Valentine *et al.* 2009).

Several precautions can help a person avoid the carotid artery when inserting a catheter into a horse's jugular vein. The following comments are made with the understanding that the site has been properly prepared for catheterization. As a matter of routine in the hospital of this case, catheters are inserted and directed caudally in the jugular vein, that is, the catheter tip is directed toward the heart. When the catheter tip is first inserted into the vein, several seconds must be allowed to elapse so that venous blood has sufficient time to travel up and flow out of the catheter thus indicating that the catheter tip is in the vein. Venous blood drips or flows slowly from the catheter's hub; it should not pulse from the catheter or flow briskly.

If there is any doubt that the catheter is in the jugular vein, it can be removed and pressure applied to the puncture site until bleeding stops, then try again. Another option once a catheter has been seated into the jugular vein, is to collect a blood sample from the catheter and analyze it with a blood gas analyzer; the PO_2 will distinguish between venous and arterial blood. As an example, during recovery of the horse of this case, blood samples were collected simultaneously from three sites: (1) the catheter in the carotid artery; (2) from the facial artery using a needle and syringe; and (3) from the catheter in the jugular vein; all samples were analyzed in the practice's clinical chemistry lab (Table 4.2). The arterial samples indicated that the horse was hypoxemic, but the arterial samples were readily distinguishable from the venous sample.

Rule-based errors relate to supervision, knowledge, training, experience, and communication. One must ask, why did the anesthetist not recognize this problem when the horse dropped to its knees after the detomidine was injected for sedation? Was there no one to advise or consult with the anesthetist on this case? Much of this scenario suggests that the anesthetist did not have adequate training in equine anesthesia, so supervision or at least the availability of assistance and advice seems inadequate. At the time of the intracarotid injection, a more senior equine clinician, some distance from the induction area, observed the horse stumble and fall, but said nothing to the anesthetist at the time, nor were questions asked as to what had happened. The system, through its silence, seems to have played a role in this error.

The fact that the horse stumbled and dropped to its knees following the injection of detomidine is a classic sign of an intracarotid injection. Since this was an elective procedure, anesthesia and surgery should have been postponed so as to give the horse time to fully recover.

During subsequent discussions of this case it was recognized that the anesthetist frequently had problems with the anesthetic management of horses although previous problems had not caused harm to horses or colleagues. It was also recognized that the anesthetist did not intentionally make errors and mistakes, and that they seemed to be due more to a lack of knowledge, training, and experience. After discussions with the anesthetist, a plan was developed to have him work closely with a more experienced equine anesthetist until an agreed-to level of competence was achieved. Although his ability to anesthetize horses improved, he was never comfortable working with them and eventually left the equine practice to work elsewhere.

Table 4.2 Results of blood gas analysis of blood samples collected simultaneously from three blood vessels in the horse during recovery and following accidental intracarotid injection of detomidine as a premedicant and ketamine plus diazepam for induction of anesthesia for laryngeal surgery. Although the horse is hypoxic, it is possible to distinguish the two arterial samples from the venous sample based on their higher P_aO_2 values.

Vessel	pH	P_aCO_2 (mmHg)	P_aO_2 (mmHg)	SBE (mEq L^{-1})
Carotid artery	7.45	57	43	+5.8
Facial artery	7.45	57	43	+5.8
Jugular vein	7.45	46	32	+7.0

SBE, standard base excess.

Near miss vignettes

Vignette 4.1

During anesthesia of a 3.5-kg domestic short-hair cat undergoing surgery for ovariohysterectomy, the anesthetist periodically sighs the cat by closing the pop-off (adjustable pressure-limiting) valve on the breathing circuit, squeezing the reservoir bag, and then opening the pop-off valve; the rest of the time the cat continues to breathe spontaneously. While sighing the cat the anesthetist is asked by the surgeon about the cat's condition. After a brief conversation the anesthetist notices that the reservoir bag is fully distended and the airway pressure is high. Fortunately the error is quickly detected and corrected without any adverse consequence to the patient.

This is a frequent error, one that has been documented a number of times in the veterinary literature (Hofmeister *et al.* 2014; Manning & Brunson 1994; McMurphy *et al.* 1995). It is so common that anesthesia machines used for human anesthesia are designed to alert anesthetists when airway pressure exceeds a preset maximum of 40 cmH$_2$O. However, veterinary anesthetists face two realities in regards to this type of error: (1) machines made for the veterinary market are not required to have this safety feature, and (2) although many veterinary practices purchase used anesthesia machines from human hospitals, these machines are frequently out of date in terms of safety features such as breathing circuit high-pressure alarms.

Possibly the most common predisposing factor for this particular error is some form of distraction; that is, some event, either internal or external to the anesthetist, occurs at the time of the ventilation maneuver and the anesthetist's attention is distracted/captured and the closed pop-off valve is temporarily forgotten. This is a slip and a short-term memory issue, thus it is a skill-based error. So, given these realities, how does one protect against this error? One possible management strategy is to develop and use the state of mind known as "mindfulness" in which the individual has a rich awareness of the work environment (Weick 2002). As such, he or she is aware of this and other potential errors and those factors that predispose to their occurrence; being aware—mindful—helps to prevent disrupting factors from occurring (see "Individual responsibility within an organization" in Chapter 2). But mindfulness depends in part on memory, a weak link in human

cognition. A more practical approach would be to provide anesthetists with a checklist that covers all items that must be in place to safely anesthetize a patient, such as the checklist developed by the Association of Veterinary Anaesthetists (see Appendix G). But checklists such as this only address checking the APL valve at the beginning of a case, but what about during case management? Again, we get back to mindfulness, but in some cases there may be mechanical fixes or forcing strategies that help us avoid such errors.

Barotrauma has been associated with the use of non-rebreathing circuits (NRB), especially in cats (Manning & Brunson 1994; McMurphy *et al.* 1995). In the cases cited by Manning the non-rebreathing circuits were attached to pop-off valves so that cats could be manually ventilated. If the anesthetist after delivering a breath to the patient, forgot to open the pop-off valve the system and reservoir bag would rapidly fill with gas and reach pressures that caused barotrauma. The faculty at Kansas State University's College of Veterinary Medicine developed a mechanical solution that prevented harm if an anesthetist forgot to open the pop-off valve (McMurphy *et al.* 1995). A positive end-expiratory pressure valve with an upper pressure limit of 15 cmH$_2$O was incorporated into the circuit so that when airway pressure exceeded that limit, the excess gas, and thus pressure, would be vented—"popped off"—and prevent barotrauma. Recognizing that we humans will err, for example, forget to open the "pop-off" valve, it becomes very clear that introducing forcing mechanisms such as this does help prevent patient harm.

Vignette 4.2

An anesthetist turns on an electronic ventilator to mechanically ventilate a patient that is hypoventilating or is apneic, but the ventilator fails to start cycling. After quickly checking the ventilator settings and connections the anesthetist discovers that the ventilator is not plugged into an electric outlet.

This is an instance where the anesthetist's mind was preoccupied with the details of setting up for the case, or with issues external to the case. It is possible that the anesthetist had a memorized checklist for setting up the anesthesia machine and ventilator prior to using them, but in the presence of distractors (internal or external), one or more "to dos" were forgotten. This is an example of Reason's lapse, one that results in an error of omission. One strategy to prevent this type of error is to attach to the anesthesia machine and ventilator an easily read and followed checklist describing how to set up the machine and ventilator and check their function, preferably prior to anesthetizing the patient; this checkout process must not be left to memory. An existing checklist that would have caught this problem before the patient was attached to the anesthesia machine and ventilator, is the United States Food and Drug Administration (FDA) Anesthesia Equipment Checkout Recommendations (see Appendix F). This checklist was current in 1993, but because of changes in the design of anesthesia machines used in human anesthesia, this universal checklist has been replaced by machine-specific checklists. Nonetheless, the FDA Anesthesia Equipment Checkout is appropriate for use in veterinary anesthesia.

A valid question at this point is, so what? The anesthetist forgot to plug in the ventilator, so what? No big deal; all he or she has to do is plug it in! This ignores an important element of distractors in error generation. If the need to ventilate the patient were to occur at the time of an emergent event, the anesthetist would be distracted and have to turn his or her attention to a piece of equipment rather than the patient; it's an unnecessary distraction that would potentially compromise patient safety.

Vignette 4.3

An anesthetist starts an infusion pump to infuse dopamine to a hypotensive patient. After 30 seconds the pump starts to alarm and reports a back-pressure error. Inspection of the intravenous setup reveals that a clip on the intravenous line designed to prevent inadvertent infusion of a drug, is clipped closed thus preventing the infusion. Unclipping the line will allow the infusion to proceed. However, a likely result is that when the clip is removed the high pressure will result in a bolus of the drug (in this case a mixed inotrope and vasopressor) being delivered to the patient and causing unintended cardiovascular effects such as hypertension and potentially a reflex bradycardia (Dr Daniel Pang, University of Calgary, personal communication, 2015).

Perhaps in such circumstances the intravenous line containing the dopamine should be disconnected prior to opening the clamp so that the bolus of drug is not administered to the patient. The line can then be reconnected and the infusion recommenced. This of course is a process that needs to be learned. As mentioned before (see Chapter 1), standardized pre-use checklists for infusion pumps do not exist. An anesthetist may have his or her own mental checklist for such devices, but an omission error is likely when relying on memory, especially in the presence of distractions.

Vignette 4.4

An arterial catheter for direct blood pressure monitoring was planned for a Yorkshire terrier dog undergoing anesthesia for abdominal surgery. Two attempts were made to insert a 25-gauge catheter into its right and left dorsal pedal arteries; both attempts failed. One catheter caused a hematoma, so gauze and an elastic wrap were placed over the site to stop the bleeding and the dog was then moved into the operating room; anesthesia and surgery lasted 3 hours. The following day the dog started to chew the foot that had the catheter-associated hematoma; subsequently a digital pad was sloughed. The presumptive diagnosis was that the hematoma and injury to the artery plus the wrap caused digital ischemia that led to tissue necrosis, hyperesthesia, and allodynia. The dog improved with time and treatment.

Two learning issues were gained from this case:

1 Any bandage applied during anesthesia to an extremity to stop bleeding must not be left in place for more than 5 minutes, a period of time sufficient in most patients to stop bleeding from a blood vessel that has been stuck with a needle or catheter.

2 A patient must not be moved into an operating room or diagnostic area with a compressive bandage on an extremity as there is a high likelihood that the bandage will be out of sight and forgotten.

In this particular case, wrapping the puncture site with elastic wrap to stop the bleeding was an acceptable plan, but it had unintended and harmful consequences in this setting and for this patient.

One strategy for avoiding this type of error is to use a specific color of elastic wrap that is broadly understood to indicate that the bandage is to be removed shortly. Alternatively, a piece of tape with "remove bandage" can be taped to the patient's head. Such direct patient labeling can also be employed for surgical procedures such as anal purse-string sutures so they are less likely to be left in postoperatively.

Vignette 4.5

A dental procedure was performed on an old terrier dog under general anesthesia. A throat pack consisting of two gauze swabs was placed into the patient's pharynx to reduce the chance of aspirating fluid or debris during the dental procedure. The table was tilted in a slightly head-down position to facilitate drainage. The dental was completed uneventfully and the isoflurane was turned off, and the dog was disconnected from the breathing system. When the dog started to swallow, the endotracheal tube was removed with the cuff partially inflated in an attempt to drag out any fluid in the airway. After extubating the dog it appeared to choke and gag. Remembering the throat pack the anesthetist, risking fingers and hand, retrieved the gauze swabs. The dog recovered without further incident.

Throat packs are simple devices used to reduce the chance of aspirating fluid or debris that may accumulate in the oropharynx during oral and nasal procedures; they are a basic device used for the safety of the patient. But, as this case demonstrates, any of our interventions have risks associated with them. In the case of dental or oral procedures the risk of a patient aspirating blood, fluid from the dental machine, or debris such as tartar or tooth fragments, is great and using a throat pack is appropriate. However, there is the risk that if accidentally left in place after extubation, the throat pack will cause a potentially fatal airway obstruction. So what forcing strategies could be used in such situations to reduce the chance that the throat pack will not be forgotten? One strategy is to make it more visible by tying a bandage "string" around the gauze swabs with the free end trailing out of the animal's mouth. But even this cuing technique may be forgotten if the anesthetist is distracted. Sticking a label to the patient as described in the previous case, is another strategy, but a better one is to link the process of removing the throat pack with extubation. One strategy is to tie one end of the bandage "string" around the gauze pack and the other to the endotracheal connector or breathing circuit so that when the patient is extubated or disconnected from the breathing system, the gauze pack is also removed. Yes, remembering to remove a pharyngeal pack at the end of a procedure is the ideal, but short-term memory and distractions are ever present and can thwart the ideal.

Vignette 4.6

A student was managing the anesthesia of a 35-kg dog undergoing a dental procedure. Midway through the procedure the dog suddenly awoke from anesthesia. Despite physical restraint, increasing vaporizer output,

and injecting propofol the animal remained very much awake. Quick inspection of the breathing system and anesthetic machine found that one end of the fresh gas hose that had been previously cut and spliced together with a five-in-one connector, had fallen off the connector and was lying on the floor; oxygen and inhalant anesthetic were not being delivered to the circle breathing system.

In the practice of this case the anesthesia machines were modified so that non-rebreathing systems, specifically Bain circuits, could be attached to the fresh gas hose thus making it possible to use the machines for anesthesia of small patients (Figure 4.2). Near the bag-end of the Bain circuit is a tapered connector to which the fresh gas line from an anesthesia machine can be attached. In this particular practice, to make this connection possible, each anesthesia machine's fresh gas hose connecting the fresh gas outlet to the machine's circle breathing circuit, was cut at its halfway point. A five-in-one connector was used to reconnect the two hose segments, one segment from the fresh gas outlet and the other from the circle breathing circuit. When a Bain circuit is used to deliver oxygen and inhalant to a small patient (<2 kg) the hose coming from the machine's fresh gas outlet is disconnected from the five-in-one connector and attached to the fresh gas connector of the Bain circuit (see Figure 4.2).

One could argue that the student anesthetist should have been more alert to this situation, but to blame the student for this error fails to recognize the nature of the system in which any student is working and learning. In a teaching hospital veterinary students are the least knowledgeable and experienced members of the medical care team. In addition, the connector and the manner in which the anesthesia machine, patient, and dental equipment were positioned in the dentistry suite placed this connector below the anesthetist's sight level. It was also discovered that the end of this particular fresh gas hose had split longitudinally so its connection to the five-in-one connector was tenuous at best.

This incident and its cause may seem unique to this particular practice, but it highlights a reality that exists in veterinary anesthesia. When equipment does not perform as we would like it to, we modify it to meet our needs, and often do so without any forethought given as to potential adverse consequences engendered by the modifications. In this case the intentionally created breaks in the fresh gas hoses of the anesthesia machines

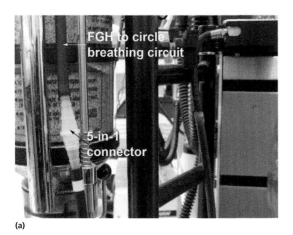

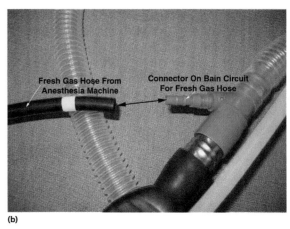

(a)　　　　　　　　　　　　　　　　　　　　　(b)

Figure 4.2 **a)** Fresh gas outlet with fresh gas hose (FGH) that is attached to the circle circuit. The hose has been cut and the two cut ends have been reconnected with a 5-in-1 connector. The hose with the yellow band that is attached to the lower end of the 5-in-1 connector, slipped off the connector and fell to the floor. Note also how cluttered this view of the machine is, a factor that made it difficult to quickly identify problems with the fresh gas hose. **b)** Bain circuit connector to which the fresh gas hose is connected.

created a hazard (a latent condition), one that went unrecognized until this error occurred. The solution that was implemented to correct this hazard was to weekly inspect all fresh gas hoses and five-in-one connectors to make sure they remained free of defects that could cause them to fail as they did in this case. This potential hazard was also made widely known within the anesthesia section so that everyone working with these machines was aware of the hazard. Of course this adds another task that has the potential to be forgotten. Including inspection of this aspect of the anesthesia machine in a pre-anesthetic checklist, one that has to be verbally "signed off" prior to anesthesia, could be a potentially better solution. However, at the end of the day, it should be remembered that anesthesia machines are built with safety in mind; modifications to them should be made cautiously and only after performing an assessment of potential risks, an assessment that recognizes the limitations of human performance.

Vignette 4.7

A 1-year-old female pygmy goat weighing 15 kg with a history of intermittent episodes of severe dyspnea, was referred to the Large Animal Hospital of the Cornell University Hospital for Animals for evaluation of a perilaryngeal mass (lymph node abscess) (Santos *et al.* 2011). The patient was scheduled for surgical excision of the mass under general anesthesia. The goat was premedicated with midazolam and ketamine, both administered IM, so as to facilitate intravenous catheterization. Once catheterized and after thorough preoxygenation, additional ketamine was administered intravenously to induce anesthesia and allow orotracheal intubation. Direct laryngoscopy revealed a large mass located cranial to the rima glottidis that caused partial obstruction of the airway and made orotracheal intubation impossible. An emergency ventral midline tracheostomy was performed and a 4.0-mm internal diameter tracheostomy tube (Crystal Trach Tube 4.0 mm; Rüsch Manufacturing (UK) Ltd, Lurgan, Co Armagh, Ireland) was inserted into the mid-cervical trachea. The capnograph showed signs of complete airway obstruction (no waveform was visible) during spontaneous breathing, and the goat could not be manually ventilated. The tracheostomy tube was removed and replaced with a new one and an appropriate carbon dioxide wave form became visible on the capnograph. Closer examination of the first tracheostomy tube revealed a complete occlusion by a plastic membrane at the level of the connector–tube interface (Figure 4.3). Although the time between tube exchanges was approximately 30 seconds, the patient's SpO_2 decreased to 87%. Once the tracheostomy tube was replaced the patient's oxygenation improved and anesthesia and surgery were completed without further complications.

Respiratory and equipment events constitute a significant source of malpractice claims (Mudumbai *et al.* 2010). Within the general category of equipment

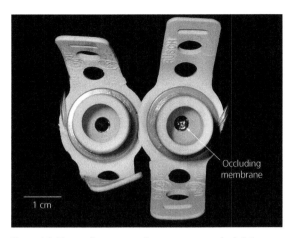

Figure 4.3 The tracheostomy tube-connector on the left is defect free while the tracheostomy tube-connector on the right is completely occluded by a plastic membrane, as indicated. From: Santos, L.C., *et al.* (2011) Tracheostomy tube occlusion during emergency tracheostomy in a pigmy goat. *Veterinary Anaesthesia & Analgesia* **38**(6): 624–625. Reprinted with permission of the publisher.

incidents, equipment misuse is three times more likely to be the cause than equipment failure (Caplan *et al.* 1997; Mudumbai *et al.* 2010). In this case, however, the tracheostomy tube, one designed for use in human patients, was defective and was the cause of this near miss. Situational awareness (Gaba *et al.* 1995) means that an anesthetist, whenever he or she uses a piece of equipment, must recognize that product flaws, although rare, may exist and must take steps to monitor a patient's response to the equipment. It is incumbent upon the anesthetist to check any piece of equipment prior to and during its use. In this case monitoring the patient with a capnograph quickly identified that the patient was not breathing through the tube and resulted in a rapid and appropriate response to this airway complication.

Vignette 4.8

In a small animal practice the veterinarian owner believed that having only one oxygen cylinder yoke on his anesthesia machine unduly limited the supply of oxygen available from the machine. To overcome this perceived limitation he removed the Pin Index Safety System pins on the machine's nitrous oxide yoke so that an additional oxygen cylinder could be used on the machine.

In error terminology this is an **intentional violation**, one performed in pursuit of what was perceived to

be a perfectly sensible goal. However, in highly defended systems a common accident scenario involves the disabling of engineered safety features (Reason 1990). In this particular example, it could be argued that as long as the pins remained on the oxygen yoke, even though they were removed from the nitrous oxide yoke, then at the very least it would not be possible to hang an inappropriate cylinder, such as nitrous oxide, on the protected oxygen yoke. But this misses two fundamental realities: (1) this action reflects a mindset that is willing to make intentional violations in order to gain some perceived benefit from the anesthesia machine, and one can only wonder what other violations have been made in the practice to achieve other ends; and (2) this violation created an error waiting to happen. We have no idea how or when an error might result from this violation, but a latent condition for error has been created.

Vignette 4.9

A horse, healthy in all respects, was undergoing general inhalant anesthesia for an orthopedic procedure. Induction and maintenance of anesthesia with controlled ventilation was uneventful until approximately 1 hour prior to the end of surgery. At that time it became difficult to maintain anesthesia in that over 30 minutes the anesthetist had to increase the isoflurane vaporizer dial setting from 2% to 4% while injecting boluses of ketamine (100–200 mg per bolus, IV) at 15-minute intervals. During this time the fresh gas flow also was increased from 5 to 7 L min^{-1} (estimated volume of the breathing circuit plus ventilator was 25 L). Despite these interventions the horse continued at a light plane throughout the remainder of anesthesia. Capillary refill time and color were normal as was rectal temperature. Results of blood gas analysis were within normal limits. Arterial blood pressure was higher than normal, but not alarmingly so given that the horse was at a light plane of anesthesia. The surgeon indicated that at this stage of the procedure there was minimal surgical stimulation. Once patient-related concerns had been ruled out the anesthetists recognized there was a problem with the anesthesia machine, but it was not possible to exchange it for another machine as one was not available.

The anesthesia machine seemed to be functioning as it should and the vaporizer's fill indicator indicated that there was sufficient volume of liquid isoflurane in the vaporizer. The drain port on the breathing circuit (which if left open can be a source of entrained room air that would dilute oxygen and inhalant anesthetic in the circuit) was checked and found to be closed. A side-stream gas analyzer was brought into the operating room and the sampling line was attached to a port on the Y-piece of the breathing circuit. Although the vaporizer was set at 4% and the fresh gas flow rate was 7 L min⁻¹ the gas analyzer gave a peak inspired isoflurane value of 1.4% and an end-tidal value of 1.2%. The vaporizer dial setting was increased to 5% (highest setting) and the

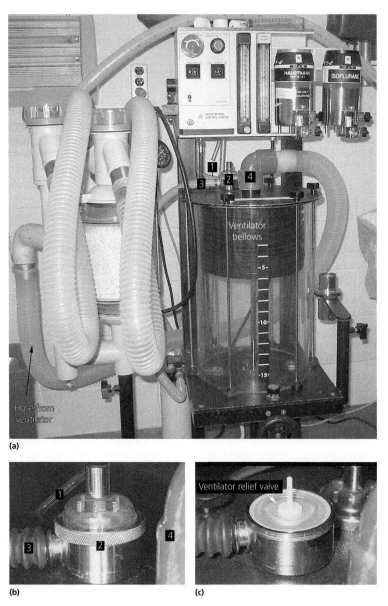

(a)

(b)

(c)

Figure 4.4 Dräger Large Animal Control Center anesthesia machine. **a)** The gas hose (1) that delivers gas to the pressure relief valve (2) shuts the valve during the inspiratory phase of mechanical ventilation. During the expiratory phase the scavenging hose (3) removes excess gas from inside the bellows, which escapes via the pressure relief valve. The ventilator hose (4) is attached to the bellows port and the other end is attached to the reservoir bag post. **b)** Close-up of the pressure relief valve on top of the ventilator bellows; same labeling as in **a. c)** Relief valve with plastic dome removed revealing silicone rubber valve.

fresh gas flow increased to 8 L min^{-1}. The effect of these interventions could not be assessed as the surgery was soon completed and the horse was moved to the recovery stall. Recovery was uneventful. Attention turned to the anesthesia machine.

The Dräger Large Animal Control Center anesthesia machine used in this case consists of a fresh gas flowmeter (oxygen), a vaporizer, breathing circuit, and an electronic time-cycled and volume-controlled ventilator (Figure 4.4). The inspiratory phase depends on a driving force of gas that fills the canister containing the bellows and compresses the bellows to generate a tidal breath that is delivered to the patient. On the top metal plate of the bellows housing are two openings, the largest of which is the outlet for the volume of gas that is delivered during inspiration from the ventilator to the patient via the ventilator hose that is connected to the reservoir bag post of the breathing circuit. The second port is much smaller and serves as the seat for a pressure relief valve that is connected to the machine's scavenging system. During inspiration a fraction of the driving gas to the bellows canister is shunted to this valve to close it so that all of the gas in the bellows is delivered to the patient and not partially evacuated through the pressure relief valve and scavenging system. The gas within the bellows consists of oxygen and inhalant anesthetic. The driving gas to the outside of the bellows is devoid of anesthetic gas.

A solution of soap and water was liberally applied to all connections related to the breathing circuit, including the breathing hoses, Y-piece, domes of the one-way flutter valves, ventilator hose, especially where it connected to the reservoir bag post and the port on the ventilator. No leaks were detected. The bellows assembly was disassembled and the bellows were filled with water to check for leaks; none were found. The pressure relief valve was then disassembled and at first glance nothing seemed amiss. Closer inspection revealed that the silicone rubber diaphragm seemed to have a defect, and when the diaphragm was gently stretched it was obvious that it was torn (Figure 4.5). During the inspiratory phase of ventilation this tear in the diaphragm allowed the driving gas to be blown into the ventilator bellows proper thus diluting the inhalant anesthetic. This problem was made known to the anesthesia section during rounds, with attention given to how to distinguish between patient-related problems and machine-related problems.

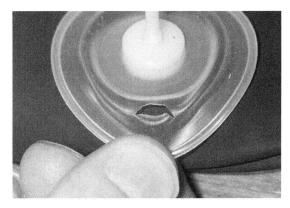

Figure 4.5 Silicone rubber diaphragm of the relief valve on the top of the bellows housing of the Dräger Large Animal Control Center anesthesia machine. During inspiration when the valve was shut by gas (oxygen) under pressure, the rip allowed fresh gas devoid of anesthetic to enter the bellows and dilute anesthetic gas in the bellows thus decreasing the concentration of anesthetic being delivered to the patient.

This case highlights the importance of having regular maintenance and servicing of anesthesia machines. Clearly it is not feasible for an anesthetist to take apart and reconstruct an anesthesia machine before every anesthetic on the off chance there may be a problem with a valve that is designed to work for many years. However, regular maintenance should be performed to ensure all of the internal workings of the machine are in good working order and are functioning properly. In this particular case, despite regular cleaning of all anesthesia machines, this problem still occurred. For the safety of anesthetized patients, be they large animals or small, and the staff working with them, when such failures occur it is important to have a back-up method (a plan) for keeping the patients anesthetized while providing oxygen and intermittent positive-pressure ventilation, such as a with-demand valve.

Conclusion

As already discussed, the incidence of equipment failure as a primary cause of errors in anesthesia, is low. But failures do occur. What is more obvious is that all too often equipment-associated problems occur as a result of human error, errors that may be minimized or avoided by appropriate education and training of staff, appropriate pre-use equipment-associated checks, and periodic maintenance of equipment.

References

Caplan, R.A., *et al.* (1997) Adverse anesthetic outcomes arising from gas delivery equipment: A closed claims analysis. *Anesthesiology* **87**(4): 741–748.

Cassidy, C.J., *et al.* (2011) Critical incident reports concerning anaesthetic equipment: Analysis of the UK National Reporting and Learning System (NRLS) data from 2006–2008. *Anaesthesia* **66**(10): 879–888.

Cooper, J.B., *et al.* (1984) An analysis of major errors and equipment failures in anesthesia management: Considerations for prevention and detection. *Anesthesiology* **60**(1): 34–42.

Fasting, S. & Gisvold, S.E. (2002) Equipment problems during anaesthesia—are they a quality problem? *British Journal of Anaesthesia* **89**(6): 825–831.

Gaba, D.M., *et al.* (1995) Situation awareness in anesthesiology. *Human Factors* **37**(1): 20–31.

Hofmeister, E.H., *et al.* (2014) Development, implementation and impact of simple patient safety interventions in a university teaching hospital. *Veterinary Anaesthesia & Analgesia* **41**(3): 243–248.

Manning, M.M. & Brunson, D.B. (1994) Barotrauma in a cat. *Journal of the American Veterinary Medical Association* **205**(1): 62–64.

McMurphy, R.M., *et al.* (1995) Modification of a nonrebreathing circuit adapter to prevent barotrauma in anesthetized patients. *Veterinary Surgery* **24**(4): 352–355.

Mehta, S.P., *et al.* (2013) Patient injuries from anesthesia gas delivery equipment: A closed claims update. *Anesthesiology* **119**(4): 788–795.

Mudumbai, S.C., *et al.* (2010) Use of medical simulation to explore equipment failures and human–machine interactions in anesthesia machine pipeline supply crossover. *Anesthesia & Analgesia* **110**(5): 1292–1296.

Reason, J.T. (1990) *Human Error.* Cambridge: Cambridge University Press.

Santos, L.C., *et al.* (2011) Tracheostomy tube occlusion during emergency tracheostomy in a pigmy goat. *Veterinary Anaesthesia and Analgesia* **38**(6): 624–625.

Singleton, R.J., *et al.* (2005) Crisis management during anaesthesia: Vascular access problems. *Quality & Safety in Health Care* **14**(3): e20–e23.

Valentine, B.A., *et al.* (2009) Cerebral injury from intracarotid injection in an alpaca (*Vicugna pacos*). *Journal of Veterinary Diagnostic Investigation* **21**(1): 149–152.

Webb, R.K., *et al.* (1993) The Australian Incident Monitoring Study. Equipment failure: An analysis of 2000 incident reports. *Anaesthesia and Intensive Care* **21**(5): 673–677.

Weick, K.E. (2002) The reduction of medical errors through mindful interdependence. In: *Medical Errors: What Do We Know? What Do We Do?* (eds M.M. Rosenthal & K.M. Sutcliffe), 1st edn. San Francisco, CA: Jossey-Bass, pp. 177–199.

CHAPTER 5

Medication Errors in Veterinary Anesthesia

> ...systemic medical errors are hard to stop because their genesis is hard to spot.
>
> *Karl E. Weick (2002)*

Medication errors are among the most commonly encountered errors in human medicine, with reports suggesting they may occur in a staggering 2–14% of all hospital admissions (Cullen *et al.* 2000; Leape 1994; Schiff & Leape 2012). They can occur in many guises and involve any part of the prescription process including choosing the drug itself, calculating the dose, writing up orders, and administering the drug. In fact preparing and administering a drug, such as an intravenous injection as part of an anaesthetic, is a surprisingly complex task involving some 30 or more steps (Woods 2005). Recognizing this complexity makes it easy to see how, when an anesthetist is under pressure or is distracted, a significant error may occur (Woods 2005).

In simple terms medication errors can be assigned to the following categories: "wrong patient," "wrong drug," "wrong dose," "wrong route," and "wrong time". However, these are just labels for a "technical error" made by an individual. By highlighting in this manner only the sharp end of the incident ignores the many system-associated conditions that set the stage for the medication error.

Literature from human medicine has provided us with most of what we know about medication errors and their root causes. But what about in veterinary medicine? In truth we really do not know the extent of the problem in veterinary medicine because there are so few data available to us (Alcott & Wong 2010; Mellanby & Herrtage 2004). Reports on medication errors have been published in a variety of journals, involving a variety of species (Alcott & Wong 2010; Kaplan *et al.* 2011; Kennedy & Smith 2014; Love *et al.* 2011; McClanahan *et al.* 1998; Means 2002; Paul *et al.* 2008; Piperisova *et al.* 2009; Smith *et al.* 1999; Wells *et al.* 2014). These articles cite the errors but their underlying causes often are not identified and the incidence in the larger patient population is unknown. In one of the only published studies to include data on the incidence of medication errors in veterinary practice, Hofmeister *et al.* found that medication error was reported in 1.2% of anesthetics prior to instituting specific error reduction strategies (Hofmeister *et al.* 2014). In that study, none of the patients died and there was little if any obvious harm to the patients, but the potential for harm was real. Unpublished data collected by the Cornell University Veterinary Medical Teaching Hospital revealed that 41 medication errors were reported over a 6-month period (see "Which incidents and errors should be analyzed?" in Chapter 3). Both of these examples involve teaching hospitals with unique environments, so the errors may seem of little relevance to general private practice. The environment of a private practice does differ from that of a teaching hospital, but despite the differences the latent conditions for medication errors are present in both. Indeed, the results of a study involving private practices for which claims were submitted to the leading veterinary indemnity insurer in the UK between January 2009 and December 2013, indicated that drug-related errors were common; the most common types of error within this category were due to incorrect choice of drug and overdose (Oxtoby *et al.* 2015). Some of the latent conditions that set the stage for medication errors are highlighted in the following cases and near miss vignettes.

Errors in Veterinary Anesthesia, First Edition. John W. Ludders and Matthew McMillan.
© 2017 John Wiley & Sons, Inc. Published 2017 by John Wiley & Sons, Inc.

Cases

Case 5.1

As preamble to the following case, we recognize that the processes described in this case are slightly historical in nature. However, we present it because it shows how system-related factors can and do set the stage for errors. The exact error described is unlikely to occur in veterinary practice today, but even now we veterinarians make modifications to processes in order to make them more efficient or economical—we describe a number of them throughout this book—and in doing so we unintentionally set in place error-generating conditions. This case also demonstrates how, if actions had been directed toward the person who seemingly caused the error as a solution to the problem, future error prevention would not have been achieved; the latent conditions that enabled the error to occur in the first place would still be present and set the system up to fail again in the future.

On a Tuesday morning a young, healthy bitch weighing 7 kg is scheduled for an ovariohysterectomy. To facilitate intravenous catheterization and induction of anesthesia she was administered acepromazine, oxymorphone, and atropine, all injected intramuscularly. Thirty minutes later she was catheterized intravenously and then anesthesia was induced with thiamylal. The catheter was flushed with heparinized saline, the trachea intubated, and the endotracheal tube was attached to a circle system to which only oxygen was delivered. A check of the patient at this time could not detect a peripheral pulse nor could heart sounds be auscultated. Cardiopulmonary resuscitation (CPR) was started promptly, but the dog did not respond to standard resuscitation efforts. An assessment of the anesthesia procedure did not reveal any clues as to the cause of death nor did a necropsy later that day.

The following day in the early afternoon a 13-kg dog scheduled for an ophthalmic procedure had a cardiac arrest several minutes after induction of anesthesia. Cardiopulmonary resuscitation was ineffective. Drug doses and procedures were in accordance with the practice's standard operating guidelines. Over the next 2 hours, two dogs and a cat were uneventfully anesthetized, but another dog weighing 6 kg and scheduled for abdominal exploratory surgery, had a cardiac arrest after intravenous catheterization and before induction of anesthesia. This dog, too, could not be resuscitated. The anesthetist reported that the dog was appropriately sedated after premedication, that its oral mucous membranes were pink and moist with a normal capillary refill time, and that its pulse was within normal parameters for rate and rhythm. According to the anesthetist the arrest occurred after the intravenous catheter had been inserted and flushed with heparinized saline.

Investigation of the incident

Inspection of the two 250 mL bottles of heparinized saline being used in the induction area revealed that, despite both bottles being clearly labeled as heparinized saline, the label on one bottle covered another label. The original label indicated that the bottle contained a potassium chloride solution (4 mmol mL^{-1}); the second label indicated the technician who had added heparin to the bottle.

Analysis of the incident

There are several questions that immediately spring to mind in this case. Was the technician responsible for the error? Was the organization—the practice—in any way responsible for the error? How could this error be prevented in the future? However, before answering these questions, contextual details are needed.

All fluids used in this practice, on both the small and large animal sides of the hospital, were made in-house at a central location because the owners believed the size of the hospital made this a cost-effective practice. For those with direct patient care responsibilities it was never clear from week to week who in the central production facility actually produced the fluids or filled orders that were submitted by the various hospital sections. Fluid volumes of one liter or less were dispensed in glass bottles with rubber stoppers and were distributed from the central location in cardboard boxes.

Every Monday and Friday, late in the afternoon, technicians throughout the hospital restocked shelves with various supplies that had been ordered earlier in the morning, including fluids. Those technicians working in sections that used heparinized saline added heparin to bottles containing 250 mL of normal saline (0.9% NaCl) to make a saline solution containing 4 units mL^{-1} of heparin. Another label was then affixed to the bottle indicating that heparin had been added, the date it was added, and by whom.

On any given day, the anesthesia service was responsible for anesthetizing 12 to 19 small animal patients, of which 80% were dogs, 15% were cats, and the remainder were birds, pocket pets, and reptiles. In this practice the anesthetic technique and drugs chosen for anesthesia were selected based on each patient's health (physical status) and the procedure to be performed. In general, anesthesia consisted of premedicating patients prior to intravenous catheterization. After the premedication drugs had taken effect a catheter was inserted into a peripheral vein, usually a cephalic vein, the catheter was capped with an injection cap, and the catheter flushed with sterile heparinized saline usually administered with a 6- or 12-mL syringe.

Prior to induction of anesthesia, each patient's heart was checked to ascertain rate and rhythm, and mucous membranes were assessed as to color and capillary refill time. Depending on the health status of each patient, anesthesia was induced with an injectable drug administered to achieve a plane of anesthesia suitable for orotracheal intubation. After intubating and securing the endotracheal tube, it would be attached to a breathing circuit, and a flow of oxygen started. At this point in the induction process the anesthetist would again check the patient's heart rate and rhythm. If the patient's condition was as expected, the anesthetist would turn on the vaporizer so as to start the delivery of inhalant anesthetic. The intravenous catheter was often flushed again at this time and then fluids were started to maintain intravascular volume during anesthesia.

Returning to the specific analysis of this case: the organization's operating procedures, specifically those for the production and delivery of fluids, created latent conditions that set the technician up as the final common pathway for this error. To the technician's credit he fully recognized his role in the error and accepted responsibility for it; there was no equivocation or attempt to place responsibility elsewhere. Of crucial importance, the technician explained how the error occurred.

Normal saline was the only fluid that had been ordered on the Monday morning prior to this incident. The technician picked up the order in its cardboard box at the central fluid production facility and took it to the anesthesia induction room. Here, as a matter of routine, every Monday and Friday afternoon, in the same location and at about the same time of day, the anesthesia technicians added heparin to bottles of normal saline to make heparinized saline. Concentrated potassium chloride was also kept in this location, but it had not been ordered that morning and the technician did not expect it to be in the box. That Monday afternoon the two

anesthesia technicians were working together to make heparinized saline, but they were having a conversation about an issue unrelated to the task at hand. This scenario describes a skill-based error due to a slip, specifically a capture slip in that the technician's attention was focused elsewhere and there was a failure of a timely check to make sure it was normal saline to which heparin was being added. It was also assumed that the box of fluids contained only normal saline because no other types of fluids had been ordered that morning. Adding heparin to normal saline was also a task performed routinely in the same familiar location twice a week.

There was no evidence that the technician intended to cause harm and the facts clearly showed that there were multiple factors that contributed to this error. In addition, the technician did not have a prior history of violations and he was intensely remorseful (see "Analysis of the person(s) at the sharp end: accountability" in Chapter 3 and Figure 3.5). Yes, the technician was responsible for the final step in the pathway to this error, but mitigating circumstances, especially the manner in which the practice made, labeled, and distributed fluids in-house (more specifically concentrated potassium chloride), and the failure at the central fluid production facility to correctly fill fluid orders, pointed to a failure of the system.

The practice owners acknowledged the mitigating factors inherent in the practice's standard operating procedures, and recognized that any person tasked with the responsibility of making up heparinized saline within the environment of this practice, was just as likely to commit the same error. No one could predict when or how such an error would occur again, but the traps—the latent conditions—were all in place waiting to generate another fluid-related error. These facts demanded a closer look at the practice's protocols and procedures concerning its fluid production and distribution processes.

As a consequence of this error, an evaluation of the system was undertaken. One immediate decision was to stop making and bottling potassium chloride solution and purchase it commercially so that there would be no chance of confusing it with normal saline. The commercial potassium chloride vials were then stocked in wards or service areas separate from all other fluids. In addition, the distinct packaging of the vials also helped prevent them from being confused with other fluids in use in the practice. For a short time the practice continued to produce normal saline and lactated Ringer's solution, especially for use in large animal patients. However, as a result of this series of adverse incidents, and because of other complaints about in-house fluids (complaints that had been ignored up to then but that were becoming more prevalent) the practice pursued an in-depth analysis of the fluid production system itself. This found that there was a lack of quality control at a number of steps in the production process. Soon thereafter the practice switched to stocking only commercially produced fluids.

A cautionary note is necessary here. Switching from in-house produced fluids to those produced commercially does not assure safe practices or patient safety. Pharmaceutical houses, in an effort to develop brand identity and market loyalty, frequently use product labeling as a marketing strategy to achieve those goals. It is not unusual for a manufacturer to produce two very different classes of drugs and label them similarly. As a result, solutions such as potassium chloride continue to be administered to human patients when the injection

of other drugs was intended (Charpiat *et al.* 2016). Figure 5.1 graphically demonstrates how similar packaging of three different types of fluids used for flushing intravenous lines or reconstituting antibiotics, can increase the likelihood that at some unknown point in time the wrong solution will be administered to a patient, possibly with fatal consequences (Lankshear *et al.* 2005).

As already mentioned, but worth repeating, had the practice approached the error as a technician-only problem and reprimanded or terminated him as the solution to the problem, there would almost certainly have been more fluid-associated patient harms or deaths at some point in the future, at a time no one could predict. However, by taking a systems approach to the problem the practice eventually discovered the root causes of this and other fluid-related problems and effectively solved the latent problems that placed all patients at risk of harm.

There is also the human side to this story. What of the technician? In a "name and shame" culture this person

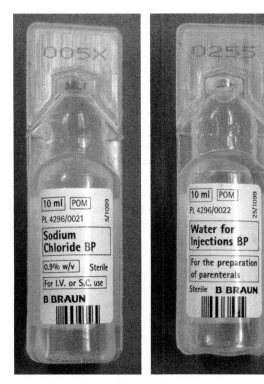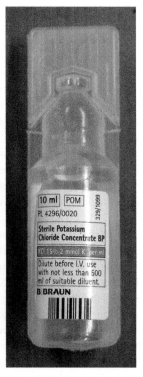

Figure 5.1 Similar packaging of various fluids used for flushing IV lines or reconstituting antibiotics, increases the likelihood that at some unknown point in time the wrong solution will be administered to a patient, possibly with fatal consequences. From: Lankshear, A.J., *et al.* (2005) *Quality and Safety in Health Care* **14**(3): 196–201. With permission of the publisher.

would have been stigmatized and chastised; at the very least their effectiveness in performing their job would have been significantly compromised. And yet this technician, by his error and full acceptance of responsibility for it, became a valuable employee. His education through this error was expensive both monetarily, emotionally, and in terms of the lives of people's pets. But from this experience he learned that it is the little details in anesthesia that can and do kill patients, an insight that was passed on to other staff in the practice.

Case 5.2

It was a busy day in a university teaching hospital. Toward the end of the day a 10-kg, 10-year-old, male, neutered terrier-cross was referred for removal of a soft tissue sarcoma and reconstruction over the hock region. It had a history of severe atopic skin disease and had been on and off corticosteroids for many years. At the time of presentation the dog was receiving 5 mg of prednisolone every other day. The animal was not easy to examine, being an itchy, snappy, and grumpy old terrier. No cardiovascular disease was evident and a chest radiograph taken by the referring veterinarian to check for metastases, revealed a normal cardiac silhouette and lung pattern. Routine blood chemistry results from a month earlier indicated a mild steroid hepatopathy.

A student assessed the patient, made a written plan, and then prepared the anesthetic. The attending anesthetist discussed the plan with the student and also performed a brief physical examination of the now decidedly annoyed dog. The odd drug choice and dosage were amended and the plan was agreed upon and finalized. The anesthetist checked the equipment and drug setup and noted that fluids had not been prepared and run through an administration set. The student was pointed in the direction of the fluid store and equipment. After discussing the patient, procedure, likely complications, and the plan with an experienced technician, the anesthetist left the area to attend to an emergency case that had just been admitted.

As per the plan, the dog was given 50 μg of medetomidine and 6 mg of methadone intramuscularly. This produced good sedation that allowed insertion of an intravenous catheter without stressing the dog, the student, or the technician! Prior to induction dexamethasone was administered intravenously. Shortly following this, anesthesia was induced with propofol and, after intubation, was maintained with isoflurane in oxygen.

Just after induction, fluids were started at 100 mL h^{-1} via a fluid pump. A peripheral nerve stimulator-guided sciatic and femoral nerve block was performed for analgesia. Capnography, pulse oximetry, indirect blood pressure via oscillometry, and electrocardiogram were monitored throughout anesthesia. Initial blood pressures were high at about 160/100 [120] mmHg (systolic/diastolic [mean] arterial blood pressure) with a heart rate of 60 beats per minute; this bradycardia was attributed to the vasoconstrictive action and reflex bradycardia associated with the medetomidine.

In the operating room, once surgery had commenced, the arterial blood pressure increased to 180/110 [130] mmHg. Initially it was assumed the nerve blocks had failed, so a bolus of fentanyl was administered and the vaporizer setting was increased. However, this made little difference. Another senior anesthetist was called in for their opinion as the initial anesthetist was still in the emergency room. As the depth of anesthesia and analgesia appeared appropriate for the surgery, the second anesthetist suggested that the hypertension might be associated with the corticosteroid administration or potentially a cuff that was too small (the circumference of the patient's leg was between two cuff sizes and the smaller cuff had been chosen as its fit was closest to ideal). As the pressure was now 190/130 [145] mmHg, acepromazine (0.1 mg) was administered intravenously. This reduced the blood pressure to the values measured at induction and the patient was managed in a mildly hypertensive state for the remaining 3 hours of anesthesia. After extubation the dog was transferred to the recovery room using a standardized communication process and hand-off sheet. Fluids were due to be continued postoperatively but stopped once the patient started to eat and drink.

The dog made a sluggish recovery and, after 45 minutes, the first anesthetist was called to the recovery room as the dog had started to develop generalized tremors. During the anesthetist's assessment the dog started to convulse with rapid progression to a grand mal seizure that responded to diazepam (5 mg IV). As the dog did not have a history of seizures a venous blood sample was drawn and analysis revealed acidosis with severe hypernatremia (185 mmol L^{-1}) and hyperchloremia.

As part of a general assessment of the patient and medications, the anesthetist checked the fluid bag and found that a bag of 7.2% sodium chloride had been hung rather than, as expected, a bag of lactated Ringer's solution or 0.9% "normal" saline. The infusion was stopped. The amount of free water necessary to reduce the dog's sodium to $150 \, mmol \, L^{-1}$ was calculated and administered over the next 4 hours. Venous blood samples were drawn and analyzed for blood gases and electrolytes every hour, tracking the sodium until it was within the reference range.

While treating the dog, every other animal in the hospital had their fluid bags checked, as was every single store of fluids. No other animals were receiving the wrong fluids, but two bags of hypertonic saline were found mixed in with the 500-mL bags of lactated Ringer's solution in the anesthesia stock (this is where the student had indicated the bag had come from when quizzed about the case). The word "quizzed" is used deliberately here; the student was not accused of wrongdoing or blamed for the error. Despite reassurances the student was found crying in the changing room later that day.

Fortunately, the dog made a complete recovery and was discharged the next day.

Investigation of the incident

So was this just a freak accident, a case of mistaken identity? Bags of one fluid look pretty similar to bags of other fluids, and to the inexperienced or distracted individual they could easily be confused. Perhaps the fluids should have been checked when they were first hung by the student and then by the attending anesthetist and technician, which was the normal routine in this teaching hospital. Also, perhaps the fluid store should have been stocked with more care and attention? Certainly, it would be easy to take this approach, emails could be sent out asking people to be more vigilant, be more careful, and the assistant who looked after the fluid store could have been reprimanded. Perhaps the problem(s) runs deeper than these frontline individuals. Let's ignore the fact that manufacturers produce drugs and fluids in almost identical packages, and focus on the systems and processes involved behind the scenes of this incident.

Interestingly, the hospital staff had recognized the potential for this type of error to occur. As a consequence hypertonic saline was not kept with other fluids. In fact, the hospital's pharmacy ordered hypertonic fluids separately and kept the stock in the pharmacy (rather in the hospital fluid store). In clinical areas of the hospital hypertonic saline was kept in separate stores and was only available in the induction area, emergency room, and ICU. In these locations it was always kept in either an emergency procedures cabinet or CRASH trolley and was clearly labeled with luminous stickers. That was what was supposed to happen.

Investigation of this incident revealed that during the previous week the last bag of hypertonic saline had been taken from pharmacy to replenish the stock in the emergency room. At that time the pharmacist had ordered a new box of ten bags from the local wholesaler. Unfortunately, on the day of delivery the pharmacist, who normally accepted and stored the bags of hypertonic saline, had taken a day's leave to care for a sick child. As a result, a technician who was busy dealing with patients, accepted delivery. The boxes of hypertonic saline, appearing identical to isotonic fluids, were then distributed throughout the hospital by a stockroom assistant (who had access to a trolley that could move large quantities of stock). In the pharmacist's absence, the assistant had been asked to restock the hospital's store of fluids as they were depleted because it had been a busy week. The boxes of fluid were stacked alongside the other fluids for later sorting.

A kennel assistant, who had been asked to get several bags of fluid for the induction room, which was running short of fluids, took the last two bags of lactated Ringer's solution from their box, and then opened the box underneath, which normally would have contained lactated Ringer's solution or at worst normal saline. The kennel assistant took three additional bags and passed them on to a student in the anesthesia unit. The student being helpful and familiar with the induction room, piled the fluid bags into the fluid cabinet. And thus a chain of events unfolded that led to the accidental administration of hypertonic saline to an anesthetised dog.

Analysis of the incident

Figure 5.2 outlines a systems walk for the process of ordering and restocking hypertonic saline in the hospital of this case. It demonstrates how the omission of one step, due to unforeseen but potentially commonplace circumstances, can set in motion a whole new cascade of unintended events that led to this error. In hindsight, it is so easy to see how this error occurred. However, at the time of the incident the preventive measures that were in place to prevent this error seemed to be perfectly adequate and working as intended.

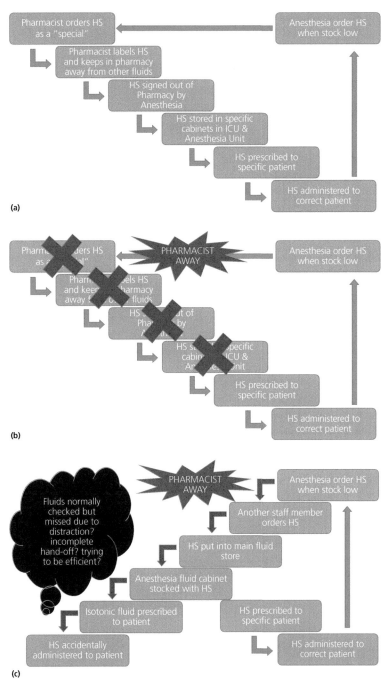

Figure 5.2 **(a–c)** Systems walk diagrams depicting the process in place for handling hypertonic saline (HS) and how unforeseen circumstances aligned to cause inadvertent infusion of hypertonic saline to a patient. **a)** The normal and expected steps of the cyclic process for ordering, procuring, handling, storing, and administering hypertonic saline in the hospital. **b)** The knock-on effects when the hospital's single pharmacist was absent. A number of critical steps in the process, including the labeling and proper distribution of hypertonic saline, did not occur. **c)** The cascade of subsequent events that led to the accidental administration of hypertonic saline to the patient of this case. The hypertonic saline had not been processed and labeled as per the hospital's standard operating procedure because the key person in the process, the pharmacist, was absent when a new supply of hypertonic saline was delivered to the hospital. When the success of a process depends on a single individual, a latent condition is potentially created that can lead to an error as occurred in this case.

The major latent conditions in this case were:

- Hypertonic saline is a rarely used "specialist" medication that was superficially identical to commonly used medications. These medications could easily be confused.
- The main barrier protecting against a potential error relied on a single individual to perform many of the key tasks (special ordering, handling, and storing of the hypertonic saline), so when that person was absent the conditions were set for an error to occur.
- Point-of-care users assumed that the upstream safeguards in place to protect against the inappropriate use of hypertonic saline were bulletproof and could not be breached.
- We often do not consider fluids to be medications and for this reason they are not treated in the same fashion as are drugs. In this hospital, fluids did not undergo the same rigorous checks as did drugs prior to their administration.

Multiple cognitive biases were also involved when hypertension was initially diagnosed during anesthesia. These included locking onto and accepting the idea that the cause was due to the long-term administration of steroid to the patient and then focusing on the size and position of the cuff as the cause of the problem. Other potential causes were not considered nor were potential biases considered such as anchoring, availability, self-satisficing, and premature closure. These biases and errors may have been influenced by:

- Having three different team members involved in the care of the case (two anesthetists and a technician), something that led to a number of unintended additional transitions in care.
- Clinicians being rushed and pulled away from anesthesia by the arrival of emergency cases.

Near miss vignettes

Vignette 5.1

Toward the end of a short anesthetic an anesthetist reaches for atipamezole to antagonize medetomidine that had been administered to the patient. For convenience the drugs are stored side by side in a drawer in the induction area. Both drugs are generic formulations consisting of clear solutions supplied in clear multi-dose vials with blue text on white labels. Instead of grabbing the atipamezole the anesthetist grabs the medetomidine and inadvertently administers additional alpha-2 sedation rather than a "reversal" agent.

Vignette 5.2

An anesthetic is planned for a cat that is to have a deep corneal ulcer and descemetocele repaired. It is a relatively straightforward case that will require the cat to receive a neuromuscular blocking agent to ensure a centrally positioned eye to facilitate the repair. The attending anesthetist fully prepares the case, checking the equipment and drawing up all drugs required for the anesthetic, including the neuromuscular blocking agent vecuronium (drawn up in a 2.5-mL syringe to facilitate multiple doses should they be required). All drugs are labeled with color-coded labels such as white labels with black text for flush, yellow labels with black text for induction agents, and so forth. Having run out of labels for neuromuscular blocking drugs (red labels with black text) the anesthetist uses a blank white label and writes "vecuronium" on it with a black-ink permanent marker. The labeled drugs are placed on a tray in the order in which they may be required: a syringe with 2.5 mL of heparinized saline for flushing the intravenous catheter, a syringe with 2.5 mL of thiopental for induction, and the syringe with 2.5 mL of vecuronium. The cat is brought to the induction room having been premedicated 30 minutes earlier with acepromazine and meperidine. The anesthetist places an intravenous catheter and reaches for and picks up the heparinized saline in the drug tray, and flushes the catheter with 1.5 mL of the solution. While reaching for the thiopental (only seconds after the catheter had been flushed) the anesthetist realizes that the catheter had been flushed with vecuronium. The calculated induction dose of thiopental is rapidly administered and the cat is intubated (slightly more easily than normal) and ventilated. The case proceeds without any further incident.

Vignette 5.3

A dog was anesthetized for a tibial plateau leveling osteotomy (TPLO) and an epidural was planned as part of the protocol. Much as for the previous case the standard procedure for inducing anesthesia involved placing all drugs (in labeled syringes) and necessary supplies on a tray, which was then taken to the induction table. In the case of this scenario cefazolin was included on the tray as it was to be administered intraoperatively. The labels for the epidural and the cefazolin were the same color: black letters on a gray background. After 5 mL of the epidural had been administered it was noticed that cefazolin was being injected and not the epidural drugs. An attempt was made to withdraw the cefazolin from the epidural space, but without success. The dog's cardiovascular and pulmonary function remained unchanged. The owners were called and told of the mistake and offered two options: wake the dog up and evaluate it for any neurological deficits, or continue with anesthesia and surgery as planned; the decision was made to wake the dog up. The dog recovered uneventfully and without neurologic dysfunction. [Permission to cite this case was generously granted by Dr Lisa Moses and Dr Andrea Looney.]

Labeling and medication errors

Labels are meant to identify drugs so that medication errors do not occur. Despite this precaution errors still occur, a reality made humorously clear by Professor Nigel Caulkett at the University of Calgary, who kindly gave us permission to present his experience with drugs, labels, and near misses:

> I distinctly remember a horse that did not go down on ketamine; it was a mini horse and I had been up for 2 nights on call. I administered a full dose of ketamine and the horse became more sedate but just stood there. I remember telling the surgery resident and anesthesia resident that I had heard of this, but never seen it. I went to grab another dose of ketamine and as I picked up the bottle I decided to check the expiry date. When I looked at the bottle, the ketamine had magically transformed itself into a bottle of Demerol [meperidine]! I used a new bottle of ketamine and the procedure went very well. Sometime later we were inducing a horse and immediately after administering the xylazine we discovered that the xylazine had transformed itself into ketamine! This was much more dramatic but luckily all [went] well. More recently I had a situation where the ketamine transformed itself into heparinized saline. This was quite boring and fixed quickly with more ketamine.
>
> I have found that if I stare at the bottle as I draw up the drug and stick a label on the syringe ASAP it usually tends to behave itself and works like it should.

Pharmaceutical houses use product labeling as a marketing strategy to achieve brand identity and consumer loyalty. As a result it is not unusual for a manufacturer to produce two very different classes of drugs and yet package them identically even with similar labels, a situation that under the right circumstances can confuse an anesthetist and result in administration of a wrong drug. For example, at any given time at the Queen's Veterinary School Hospital, University of Cambridge, there are often six or more drugs commonly administered during the peri-anesthetic period that are transparent solutions, in clear multi-use 10-mL vials, with white labels and blue text. Under these conditions the only barrier to error is vigilance, a fallible error prevention strategy.

When our level of activation is either too low (too few demands, boredom, fatigue) or too high (excessive demands, stress, and pressure), the human information search function becomes coarser, and fewer clues are considered for the information being processed (Hubler *et al.* 2014). Even when conflicting information—such as an incorrect medication label—is present, the view that conforms to the current expectation—"I'm using the correct drug"—will be projected onto the variant form of reality (Hubler *et al.* 2014). In other words, we are likely to see what we want to see rather than what really is.

One study has shown that if an incorrect drug is drawn up, there is an 81% chance it will actually be administered to a patient (Currie *et al.* 1993; Jensen *et al.* 2004). If the incorrect drug is in a properly labeled syringe, there is a 93% chance it will be administered (Currie *et al.* 1993). It has been suggested that this type of error is a slip, which occurs when the anesthetist is on "automatic pilot" and distracting factors are at play, such as fatigue, haste, and inattention (Currie *et al.* 1993). With all of these thoughts in mind about medication errors, one fact seems to be a recurring preventive strategy: read the label before administering a drug to a patient (Currie *et al.* 1993; Jensen *et al.* 2004). However, in the heat of the moment this is easier said than done!

Faulty labeling (applying an incorrect sticky label to a syringe) is a contributing factor to medication errors. A variety of label colors are meant to help anesthetists discern one type of drug from another, but using color either for a label's background or text as a method of drug identification is fraught with problems. It is not unusual for two completely different drugs to have similar labels. Add in other factors that can affect our ability to discriminate one color from another, such as lighting-related issues, shades of color, fatigue, and so forth, and it becomes obvious that color as a means of identifying medications may not be as foolproof as we would like. Other techniques need to be used, such as applying a label for an injectable drug to both needle cap and syringe; this helps to **force** the caregiver to check the label (**a forcing technique**) when removing the needle cap. However, sticking a label to both needle cap and syringe adds another step to the process, one that may be easily forgotten when an anesthetist is pressed for time, distracted, or tired.

Similarity of packaging and product labels poses problems when multiple drugs are stored in close proximity to each other, a frequent practice strategy meant to aid efficiency as drugs are often administered together or are required in urgent circumstances. No one wants to run to several separate cabinets gathering drugs needed for a basic case or, even more critically, during an emergency. But the reality of medication packaging and the practice of storing different drugs in close proximity to each other create the conditions for a medication error.

A human factors solution to this problem would be to change how anesthetics are prepared so as to lessen the chance of medication errors such as syringe swaps. One strategy is to only draw up drugs that will be required immediately or required in an emergency. All other drugs can be kept separately and still in their vials, often in separate trays. For example, in equine anesthesia at the Cambridge Equine Hospital, University of Cambridge, premedicants are kept in one tray, induction drugs in another, and heparinized saline in a third. Requiring an anesthetist to draw up a drug out of a vial just before administering it, rather than having it readily available in a syringe, provides anchoring and a natural pause point that is more likely to capture and force the anesthetist's attention to the label. However this may cause a delay so may not be ideal for drugs likely to be needed in an emergency situation.

Vignette 5.4

A 1.5-kg Chihuahua is being managed following surgery to correct a luxating patella. For analgesia it is to receive 0.5 mg of morphine (10 mg mL^{-1}) for a total volume of 0.05 mL to be slowly injected intravenously as the dog is difficult to inject intramuscularly. The drug is drawn up into a 1-mL syringe, and to facilitate slow administration it is diluted to a volume of 1 mL with normal saline. The drug is administered by an intern over 10 minutes as per the instructions and all goes well. The intern moves onto administering treatments to other patients in the ward. Ten minutes later the intern notices that the dog is unconscious, it is cold with

a slow respiratory rate and significant bradycardia (heart rate of 30 beats per minute). The on-call anesthetist is called and opioid overdose is diagnosed as the likely cause. Naloxone is titrated to effect and the dog recovers. A quick investigation of the incident reveals the cause. The morphine had been drawn up into the syringe correctly, but when diluting the drug the 0.1 mL dead space of the syringe and needle had not been accounted for. Consequently, an additional 0.1 mL (1 mg) of morphine had been drawn up into the syringe and administered to the patient, a dose equivalent to a three-times overdose.

This is an example of a medication error in which the correct dose was calculated, the method of administration was appropriate, but an error occurred during the preparation stage. This type of error is probably more common than we think. Whenever we combine and mix drugs in the same syringe the volume of the dead space within the syringe and needle alters the amount of the first drug that is drawn up. When administering larger volumes such inaccuracies are negligible and for many drugs their dosing range and safety margin are so wide as to pose little risk to the patient. But, in some circumstances, these small discrepancies in volume can be important.

> Remembering when, as a resident, I (MWM) started using low doses of medetomidine plus an opioid for premedicating patients and I thought how effective 20 μg (total dose) of medetomidine was in sedating the average 4-kg cat. This was until a colleague asked me, "How come it works for you and not for me?" Initially I attributed the efficacy to my superior cat whispering skills, but it soon became apparent that I was drawing up the medetomidine first and she was drawing up the opioid first. The dead space in the syringes and needles I was using added about 50 μg of medetomidine into the mix that I drew up!

A number of methods can be employed to reduce the problem with syringe and needle dead space, including:
- The use of low dead space syringes when administering small volumes.
- First draw up drugs with larger dosing ranges or margins of safety followed by those drugs with smaller dosing ranges or margins of safety.
- When diluting drugs with saline, first draw up a small volume of saline to fill the dead space of the syringe prior to drawing up the primary drug(s). This can be assisted by writing clear instructions that list the order in which the drugs are to be drawn up into the syringe.

All of these suggested precautions have to be learned and then used over and over again to become habits, a reality that makes medication errors some of the most difficult of error types to reduce.

Conclusions

These examples of medication errors highlight some of the latent conditions that make these types of errors possible in veterinary anesthesia. These few examples also show that medication errors are not simply due to the individual administering the drug, the drug itself, or the labeling. There are obviously multiple causes underlying each of these errors, a reality strongly suggesting that when an initial analysis of a medication error seems to identify an individual or a few factors as the cause of the error, further, deeper analysis is necessary. Doing so invariably reveals significant latent factors that may have been missed but that set the stage for these errors. Complacency with the system and saying "We've always done it this way and never had a problem as we are vigilant" does not stop bad stuff from happening. Even when systems are put in place to avoid errors, conditions sometimes align, defences are breached, and errors occur.

References

Alcott, C.J. & Wong, D.M. (2010) Anaphylaxis and systemic inflammatory response syndrome induced by inadvertent intravenous administration of mare's milk in a neonatal foal. *Journal of Veterinary Emergency and Critical Care (San Antonio, Tex.: 2001)* **20**(6): 616–622.

Charpiat, B., Magdinier, C., Leboucher, G., & Aubrun, F. (2016) Medication errors with concentrated potassium intravenous solutions: Data of the literature, context and prevention. *Annales Pharmaceutiques Françaises* **74**(1): 3–11.

Cullen, D.J., *et al.* (2000) Prevention of adverse drug events: A decade of progress in patient safety. *Journal of Clinical Anesthesia* **12**(8): 600–614.

Currie, M., *et al.* (1993) The Australian Incident Monitoring Study. the "wrong drug" problem in anaesthesia: An analysis of 2000 incident reports. *Anaesthesia and Intensive Care* **21**(5): 596–601.

Hofmeister, E.H., *et al.* (2014) Development, implementation and impact of simple patient safety interventions in a university teaching hospital. *Veterinary Anaesthesia & Analgesia* **41**(3): 243–248.

Hubler, M., Koch, T., & Domino, K.B. (eds) (2014) *Complications and Mishaps in Anesthesia*. Berlin: Springer.

Jensen, L.S., *et al.* (2004) Evidence-based strategies for preventing drug administration errors during anaesthesia. *Anaesthesia* **59**(5): 493–504.

Kaplan, M.I., *et al.* (2011) Adverse effects associated with inadvertent intravenous penicillin G procaine-penicillin G benzathine administration in two dogs and a cat. *Journal of the American Veterinary Medical Association* **238**(4): 507–510.

Kennedy, M.J. & Smith, L.J. (2014) Anesthesia case of the month. Accidental lidocaine overdose during surgery for vertebral fractures. *Journal of the American Veterinary Medical Association* **245**(10): 1098–1101.

Lankshear, A.J., *et al.* (2005) Evaluation of the implementation of the alert issued by the UK National Patient Safety Agency on the storage and handling of potassium chloride concentrate solution. *Quality and Safety in Health Care* **14**(3): 196–201.

Leape, L.L. (1994) Error in medicine. *Journal of the American Medical Association* **272**(23): 1851–1857.

Love, D.C., *et al.* (2011) Dose imprecision and resistance: Free-choice medicated feeds in industrial food animal production in the United States. *Environmental Health Perspectives* **119**(3): 279–283.

McClanahan, S., *et al.* (1998) Propylene glycol toxicosis in a mare. *Veterinary and Human Toxicology* **40**(5): 294–296.

Means, C. (2002) Selected herbal hazards. *Veterinary Clinics of North America Small Animal Practice* **32**(2): 367–382.

Mellanby, R.J. & Herrtage, M.E. (2004) Survey of mistakes made by recent veterinary graduates. *Veterinary Record* **155**(24): 761–765.

Oxtoby, C., *et al.* (2015) We need to talk about error: Causes and types of error in veterinary practice. *Veterinary Record* **177**(17): 438–445.

Paul, A.L., *et al.* (2008) Aplastic anemia in two kittens following a prescription error. *Journal of the American Animal Hospital Association* **44**(1): 25–31.

Piperisova, I., *et al.* (2009) What is your diagnosis? Marked hyperchloremia in a dog. *Veterinary Clinical Pathology/American Society for Veterinary Clinical Pathology* **38**(3): 411–414.

Schiff, G.D. & Leape, L.L. (2012) Commentary: How can we make diagnosis safer? *Academic Medicine* **87**(2): 135–138.

Smith, B.I., *et al.* (1999) Selenium toxicosis in a flock of Katahdin hair sheep. *Canadian Veterinary Journal* **40**(3): 192–194.

Weick, K.E. (2002) The reduction of medical errors through mindful interdependence. In: *Medical Errors: What Do We Know? What Do We Do?* (eds M.M. Rosenthal & K.M. Sutcliffe), 1st edn. San Francisco, CA: Jossey-Bass, pp. 177–199.

Wells, J.E., *et al.* (2014) Cyclophosphamide intoxication because of pharmacy error in two dogs. *Journal of the American Veterinary Medical Association* **245**(2): 222–226.

Woods, I. (2005) Making errors: Admitting them and learning from them. *Anaesthesia* **60**(3): 215–217.

CHAPTER 6

Errors of Clinical Reasoning and Decision-making in Veterinary Anesthesia

What we observe is not nature in itself but nature exposed to our method of questioning.
Werner Heisenberg, Physics and Philosophy (Penguin Classics, 2000)

Removing the stigma of bias clears the way toward accepting the capricious nature of decision making, and perhaps goes some way toward exculpating clinicians when their diagnoses fail.
Pat Croskerry (2003)

Clinical reasoning and decision-making are critical skills in all areas of medicine including anesthesia. They allow clinicians to efficiently and effectively make a diagnosis and establish a treatment plan. In doing so, information must be gathered from multiple sources, sorted, assimilated, and then formed as a coherent narrative or pattern so that the information makes sense. This information must be cross-referenced against knowledge pertaining to physiological and pathophysiological processes so a diagnosis can be made and treatments chosen.

For some complications encountered during anesthesia the diagnosis (cause) and treatment (intervention) are clear; the complication is straightforward and requires little more than pattern matching, memory, and action. For example, bradycardia following the administration of a potent opioid is a known side effect, one that is easily treated by the administration of an anticholinergic drug such as atropine or glycopyrrolate. These skills derive from the anesthetist's education, training, experience and, to a certain extent, the amount of preparation and planning that has gone into the anesthetic protocol. The latter two factors—preparation and planning—are important as many complications can be predicted and specific monitoring and interventions strategies can be set in place even before any anesthetic drugs have been administered. However, where there is doubt and uncertainty about a diagnosis there is a requirement for clinical reasoning and decision-making.

Anesthetists face some unique stresses in the process of making clinical decisions, especially when dealing with anesthetic complications. The acute and sometimes immediately life-threatening nature of anesthetic complications impose real and significant pressures of time upon anesthetists to identify the cause of a problem and select and institute an appropriate intervention(s). But the manner in which an anesthetist's thought processes develop in response to clinical information, typically acquired through their senses and an array of monitoring equipment, can be easily influenced by a variety of external and internal factors (Croskerry 2013; Reason 2004) that make these processes vulnerable to error.

The diagnostic process has been extensively studied and reported on in the literature, probably because it is the foundation of medical practice (Croskerry 2005). Many cognitive factors influence how diagnoses are made, and the summation of their effects result in an action consisting of a diagnosis and plan for intervention (treatment). According to Croskerry, the action can take one of three decision outcome modes (Croskerry 2005):

- **Flesh and Blood** decisions represent "practical decision-making" wherein the clinician is aware of ever present time pressures and resource availability, where decisions are made expeditiously and often with an incomplete clinical picture (partial physiological data or diagnostic tests). The clinician uses clinical intuition, pattern matching and a "best guess" approach to make a presumptive diagnosis.

Errors in Veterinary Anesthesia, First Edition. John W. Ludders and Matthew McMillan.
© 2017 John Wiley & Sons, Inc. Published 2017 by John Wiley & Sons, Inc.

- The **Casablanca**[1] **Strategy** aims to delay making a decision until a later time. Such a strategy of "buying time" has merit in that it stems from the recognition that some conditions, although seemingly acute and serious, can spontaneously resolve with a "tincture of time." In anesthesia this outcome style serves multiple purposes. Firstly, many problems in anesthesia are short-lived, transient, and self-limiting and require little or no intervention thus avoiding unnecessary interventions with their inherent risks. Secondly, it allows detachment from the intuitive mode of thinking, thus providing an opportunity for reflection, analysis, and other ideas to develop. Thirdly, the strategy keeps the anesthetist busy, generating a sense of something being done. Finally, time is allowed for events to develop or further define themselves in a clearer fashion.
- The **Formal Work-Up** results when the acuity and diagnostic hypothesis are clearer. True, the initial response may have been broad in scope and made to stabilize a patient, but the subsequent formal investigation, consisting of iterative hypothesis testing and refinement of differential diagnoses, progresses until a definitive diagnosis is made.

The correct decision-making style must be matched to the clinical situation for appropriate care to be delivered to the patient. Good clinical judgment can be defined as a clinician's ability to choose the appropriate decision-making style in any given situation. Diagnostic errors, on the other hand, are those errors caused by faulty clinical reasoning or decision-making, for instance, when a diagnosis is unintentionally delayed (sufficient information was available earlier), a diagnosis is wrong (another diagnosis was made before the correct one), or a diagnosis is missed (no diagnosis was ever made) (Balla *et al.* 2012).

Specific data on diagnostic error in anesthesia are not readily available. However, depending on the specialty in human medicine, diagnostic errors may account for up to 20% of in-hospital patient deaths (Graber *et al.* 2005; Graber 2013). Graber identified cognitive factors as accounting for 58% of diagnostic errors, while organizational factors account for 39%, and technical factors for only 3% (Graber *et al.* 2005). It is important to note that cognitive factors alone or when combined with organizational factors, have a greater impact on patients than do organizational factors by themselves (Graber *et al.* 2005).

A study of claims submitted to the leading veterinary indemnity insurer in the UK indicates that cognitive limitations were an important source of error in individual clinicians, with slips and lapses identified as the most frequent types of errors (Oxtoby *et al.* 2015). Indeed, the bulk of the human medical literature suggests that most diagnostic errors are cognitive in origin, occurring in the intuitive mode of cognitive processing and as a consequence of one or more cognitive biases (Norman & Eva 2010). Croskerry (2003) compiled and defined the most comprehensive list of heuristics and cognitive biases pertaining to diagnostic error to date.[2] This list was refined by Stiegler *et al.* (2012) to create a catalogue of anesthesia-specific cognitive errors. These biases are outlined under "Pattern matching and biases" in Chapter 2, and we often refer to them in the following cases and near miss vignettes.

Cases

Case 6.1

A young male polar bear weighing 318 kg was housed in a zoological exhibit that used a 6 m deep moat to separate observers from the observed. The bear was housed with a female polar bear, and he had a habit of jumping on her when she least expected it. The bear's problems started one early spring day when he tried to jump on the female as she was walking close to the moat's edge. The female saw the start of his jump and, having grown tired of these male shenanigans, she ducked; the bear became airborne (albeit briefly) and flew over her and down into the moat.

---

[1] According to Croskerry, the term is taken from the dialogue in the closing scene of the 1942 Warner Bros movie "Casablanca," in which the police chief gives an order to "round up the usual suspects," so as to gain some time despite already suspecting who the culprit is. The term was first used by Croskerry and staff at the Emergency Department of Dartmouth General Hospital to describe the blood work required for various workups: Casablanca 1 referred to a small panel, and Casablanca 2 to a large panel of usual suspects.

[2] Croskerry uses the term "Cognitive Dispositions to Respond" (CDR) to describe these psychological factors, including terms such as heuristics, cognitive biases, failure, and error, so as to avoid the negative connotation associated with these terms.

Remote examination of the bear in the moat confirmed that his hindlegs were fractured, but he was alert and attentive. Although housed in a zoo he was a dangerous animal, which made it impossible to physically examine him more thoroughly at that point in time. The attending veterinarian, recognizing that the bear's nature precluded a full examination, was rightfully concerned about internal injuries. It was assumed that the bear would not eat if there were significant internal injuries, so he was offered an apple which he promptly ate, evidence confirming that the bear did not have internal injuries. The bear was scheduled for an orthopedic examination and possible surgery the following day at a tertiary care facility. As often happens with zoo-related events, the press and public were keenly interested in the bear's condition and his surgical management.

At the tertiary care facility the bear was lightly anesthetized with etorphine and xylazine delivered via a pole syringe. Forty minutes later he was removed from the cage and masked to a deeper plane of anesthesia with halothane in oxygen delivered from a large-animal anesthesia machine. During induction a concern was expressed about the bear's thick fur and the possibility that he would develop hyperthermia during anesthesia. After 10 minutes of mask induction the bear was intubated and the endotracheal tube was attached to the breathing circuit. Because of concerns about etorphine-induced hypoventilation, intermittent positive pressure ventilation was started at 5 breaths per min. After about 30 minutes the vaporizer dial setting was turned down.

Radiographs (Figure 6.1) showed that the right tibia had a complete mid-shaft fracture and the distal end of the left femur was fractured. A team of orthopedic surgeons believed the fractures were repairable and the bear was prepared for surgery.

During this time the bear was instrumented for physiological monitoring and a lingual arterial blood sample was obtained for hematocrit (44%), total solids (6.5 g dL^{-1}), and blood gas analysis (pH 7.40, P_aCO_2 49 mmHg, P_aO_2 174 mmHg, and base balance +5.2 mEq L^{-1}). The electrocardiogram showed a sinus tachycardia (150 beats per minute), and a temperature probe inserted via the esophagus to the level of the heart, indicated a body temperature of 39.5 °C. The tachycardia was attributed to both the slightly elevated P_aCO_2 and the hyperthermia, which in turn was attributed to the hospital's warm environment and the bear's dense fur coat. Once the bear was moved into the operating theater, a catheter was inserted into a lingual artery for monitoring blood pressure and sampling arterial blood for blood gas analysis. Throughout anesthesia the mean arterial blood pressure ranged from an initial high of 153 mmHg to a low of 72 mmHg with the majority of readings between 100 and 110 mmHg. Four arterial blood samples subsequently collected over the course of 4 hours of anesthesia showed an average P_aO_2 of 470 mmHg (range: 445–491 mmHg); an average P_aCO_2 of 45 mmHg for the first 3 hours of anesthesia and an average of 28 mmHg (range: 26–30 mmHg) for the fourth hour of anesthesia; base balance averaged +5.8 mEq L^{-1} (range: +5.2 to +6.5 mEq L^{-1}). During the

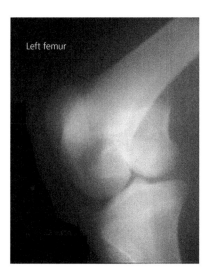
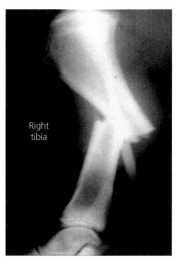

Figure 6.1 Leg fractures in a polar bear. Radiograph on the left is of the left femur showing a fracture of the distal end of the femur. The radiograph on the right shows a mid-shaft fracture of the right tibia.

last two hours of anesthesia the bear was breathing spontaneously and hyperventilating, a response attributed to hyperthermia. Body temperature, which had increased from 39.5 °C to 41.1 °C, had decreased to 40 °C and remained at that temperature throughout the remainder of anesthesia. This decrease in temperature was a result of packing ice around the bear's chest and forelimbs and eventually around the breathing circuit. At one point during anesthesia the anesthetist noted that the abdomen seemed "fluidy," but no further observations were made or actions taken.

The surgery was completed within 5 hours and anesthesia was stopped soon thereafter. The bear was given an analgesic, transferred to his cage, and given diprenorphine (M50-50) to reverse any remaining effects of the etorphine; he seemed to be recovering as expected. Approximately one hour later the bear died while being transported to the zoo. At necropsy the bear was found to have a ruptured stomach and a complete diaphragmatic hernia (Figure 6.2).

Initial analysis of the case

The referring veterinarian, a well-respected, knowledgeable, and competent zoo veterinarian, explained to the anesthesia and surgical team his thought processes and diagnostic approach to evaluating this polar bear's injuries. Even though the bear was seriously injured, he was still a very dangerous animal, a fact that made hands-on physical examination impractical. The feeding of the apple to the bear seemed like a reasonable

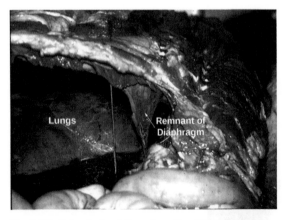

Figure 6.2 Abdominal and thoracic cavity of the polar bear at necropsy. View is from the cranial abdominal cavity toward the ruptured diaphragm and open thoracic cavity. A remnant of the diaphragm is hanging from the thoracic wall.

approach to determine if internal injuries existed. After all, what animal with serious internal injuries would eat? For the anesthesia and surgical team to question this assessment and conclusions of the zoo veterinarian did not seem collegial as he had more experience with zoo species than they did. Questioning his diagnostic approach and conclusions seemed to imply, at least in the collective mind of the team at the time, that they were questioning his medical competency. This mindset, of course, is exactly what Reason cautions against: professional courtesy must not get in the way of checking colleagues' knowledge and experience, particularly when they are strangers (Reason 2004).

The error in this case was two-fold: (1) failure to request a more thorough physical examination of the bear for fear of offending the zoo veterinarian or at least seeming to be uncollegial; and (2) assuming there were barriers, whether real or imagined, to doing a more thorough medical examination. After all, once the bear was anesthetized, all concerns about examining a dangerous animal were moot and all barriers to performing a thorough physical examination were removed. But other biases and perceived barriers persisted in the minds of the team members, but these were never openly discussed.

Investigation of the case

The circumstances surrounding this case, the context in which it occurred but not mentioned in the case presentation, explain many of the biases that set the stage for the errors in decision-making that were the basis of this diagnostic error. Some of the factors were non-medical in nature and external to the practice but significantly affected the management of this patient. There were also patient-related factors.

A perceived barrier to conducting more diagnostic techniques was that a definitive diagnosis had already been made (premature closure), and the admonition that none of the bear's fur was to be clipped for minor techniques, such as needle aspirates of the abdominal cavity, until it was determined if the fractures could be repaired. Once it was decided that the fractures could be repaired, other diagnostic tests became irrelevant in the minds of the team members because other injuries were no longer considered; attention was focused (coning of attention) on surgical repair of the fractures.

Soon after the bear was injured the local press picked up on his condition and closely followed his progress.

Thus the team came to believe that there was a great deal of pressure to present as positive a picture as possible concerning the bear's condition and surgical management. In addition, it had been made clear to the team that if the fractures could not be repaired, the bear would be euthanized and its body prepared for public display. No member of the team wanted to euthanize the bear, one that the public knew and loved; as one team member stated, "Who wants to euthanize a bear with a name?" Although euthanasia is a humane procedure, one that is performed by veterinarians for the best of medical reasons, not infrequently it is viewed as a sign of failure. In this particular case none of the team members wanted to be the veterinarian recommending euthanasia of the bear. As a result, there developed a "can do" attitude amongst team members in terms of the bear's surgical management. This mindset created blinders—tunnel vision—on the team's thinking and made it difficult for them to consider options other than repairing the fractures.

There were two other subtle influences on the anesthesia and surgery team regarding euthanasia. Public sentiment surrounding the creation of this teaching hospital a few years previously was best described as polarized; many supported and many opposed its creation. This led to a perception, whether real or not, that the teaching hospital was under public scrutiny, especially by the state's legislature.

The teaching hospital was a short walk from a large regional medical center. One day while waiting in the lunch line at the medical center, two surgical nurses were overheard commenting on how stupid veterinarians were because they did not know that fractured bones in horses could be repaired. This conversation was prompted by a recent on-track euthanasia of a race horse that had fractured its leg during a race. These were subtle but real influences on the team members, influences that contributed to a mindset that considered euthanasia as a sign of failure.

Obviously this bear was a wild animal and in its normal habitat it would be a predator. How might this reality affect its management? The assumption that the bear would not eat the offered apple if it had severe internal injuries failed to consider the nature of the animal. There is no survival advantage for a predator to show signs of disease, for by doing so the predator becomes prey. This reality of the animal's natural behavior was not considered by members of the team.

To summarize, there were several factors that prevented the entire team from correctly identifying the extent of this bear's injuries:

- Failure to question a colleague's assessment and diagnosis of the bear's condition.
- A bias that euthanasia of the bear would be viewed by many, especially the public, as a sign of failure.
- An assumption that various findings such as tachycardia and hyperthermia were due to the unique nature of the bear when in fact these findings were easily explained by less exotic considerations attributable to the trauma, such as peritonitis and fever.
- Holding on to admonitions about how the bear was to be managed long after the justifications for those admonitions had passed.

The bear died as a result of undiagnosed and untreated severe internal injuries. Had these injuries been diagnosed at presentation to the tertiary care facility, the bear would have been promptly euthanized. This, of course, was the one thing everyone wanted to avoid, but which would have been the most medically sound management of the bear. The chances of surgically and medically managing the bear's fractures and internal injuries were nil; it was a wild animal and the type of intensive hands-on care he would have required postoperatively was neither feasible nor safe.

Case 6.2

A 5-month-old 4-kg male Shetland sheepdog was referred to a veterinary teaching hospital because of hindlimb paralysis that was unresponsive to treatment with steroids. Two days previously, the owners' child had been playing roughly with the dog just prior to the onset of paralysis.

Initial examination revealed a bright and alert young dog with paralysis of both hindlimbs. Heart and respiratory rates were 84 beats per minute and 24 breaths per minute, respectively; rectal temperature was 38.5 °C, hematocrit (Hct) 34%, and plasma total protein concentration $50\,g\,L^{-1}$. Lateral and ventrodorsal radiographic views of the vertebral column revealed that the caudal end of lumbar vertebra 5 (L5) was fractured and the distal fragment and vertebral column were displaced cranially and laterally to the left thus fully compromising the neural canal (Figure 6.3). There was no evidence of free fluid in the abdominal cavity. With the owners' informed consent, the dog was anesthetized for surgical reduction and stabilization of the fracture.

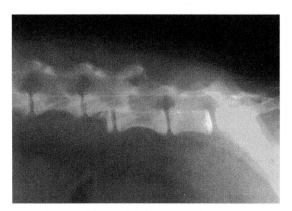

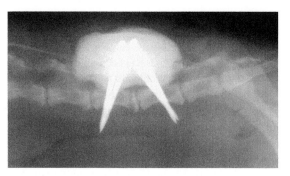

Figure 6.4 Lateral radiograph showing reduction and fixation of the vertebral fracture in the 5-month-old 4-kg male Shetland sheepdog. Reused from: Ludders, J.W., *et al.* (1998) Anesthesia case of the month. *Journal of the American Veterinary Medical Association* **213**(5): 612–614. With permission of the publisher.

Figure 6.3 Lateral radiograph of the spine of the 5-month-old 4-kg male Shetland sheepdog. The fracture is at the caudal end of L5 with the distal fragment and vertebral column displaced cranially and laterally to the left of midline; the neural canal is fully compromised in that it is not aligned. Reused from: Ludders, J.W., *et al.* (1998) Anesthesia case of the month. *Journal of the American Veterinary Medical Association* **213**(5): 612–614. With permission of the publisher.

The dog was catheterized intravenously in the ICU and subsequently premedicated by an anesthesia resident with diazepam, butorphanol, and glycopyrrolate, all given intravenously. After premedicating the dog it was anesthetized with thiamylal, intubated, started on isoflurane (1.2%) in oxygen (2 L min⁻¹) and allowed to breathe spontaneously. The dog was monitored with an electrocardiogram, and systolic arterial blood pressure was indirectly measured and recorded using a Doppler device (Model 811b; Parks Medical Electronics Inc., Aloha, OR, USA) with its probe placed over the plantar common digital artery and the cuff placed around the leg above the hock and attached to a sphygmomanometer.

At induction, the dog's heart rate was 143 beats per minute and systolic blood pressure was 110 mmHg. Throughout the 3 hours of surgery, the heart rate fluctuated between 100 and 170 beats per minute, and systolic arterial blood pressure fluctuated between 100 and 140 mmHg. The isoflurane vaporizer setting varied from 1.0 to 1.5% during anesthesia, and nitrous oxide (50%) was used to supplement isoflurane. Vecuronium bromide (a neuromuscular blocking drug) was administered to provide muscle paralysis and facilitate surgical reduction of the fracture. During the following 2 hours ventilation was controlled with a mechanical ventilator at 11 breaths per minute. Methylprednisolone sodium

succinate and cefazolin were given at 50 and 120 minutes, respectively, after the start of anesthesia.

While the surgeon was stabilizing the fracture with Steinmann pins, the Doppler's audible signal (indicating the flow of blood through the artery) stopped and could not be re-established even after the location and position of the probe were checked and adjusted on the hindleg. Another Doppler device was obtained, its probe was placed over the dog's palmar common digital artery, and a strong signal was obtained; surgery and anesthesia continued for another hour.

Near the end of surgery the dog was prepared for transport from the operating room to radiology. Nitrous oxide was discontinued 10 minutes before transport and the dog was weaned from the ventilator. For most of the anesthetic period, the dog was judged to be at a moderate plane of anesthesia. However, while preparing the dog for transport and during radiography, the dog was judged to be at a lighter plane of anesthesia based on increases in systolic arterial blood pressure (from 110 to 140 mmHg) and respiratory rate (from 12 to 15 breaths per min). To maintain an adequate plane of anesthesia, the isoflurane vaporizer dial setting was increased from 0.9% to 1.5%. The radiographs showed good reduction and alignment of the fracture (Figure 6.4).

To make recovery smoother, the dog was given butorphanol for analgesia and diazepam for muscle relaxation and tranquilization. As the dog recovered from anesthesia, it appeared uncomfortable in that it whined and looked at its hindquarters. Twenty-five minutes later, oxymorphone and acepromazine were given, both intravenously, because the dog seemed more painful and anxious. Despite these drugs, the dog continued seemingly to be uncomfortable and to focus its attention on its hindquarters. At this time the mucous membranes of the penis were noticed to be pale. In general, recovery was not progressing as expected.

While in the radiology suite and then in the recovery room, evaluation of the postoperative radiographs raised questions amongst the anesthesia-surgical team members about the possibility of one or more Steinmann pins affecting blood flow to the hindquarters, specifically flow through the abdominal aorta.

Pulses in the femoral and dorsal pedal arteries could not be palpated. Application of a Doppler probe to either pedal artery did not yield an audible blood-flow signal, but a signal was detected when the probe was placed over a palmar common digital artery in a forelimb. On the basis of these findings and the dog's behavior, it was re-anesthetized for surgical exploration of its abdomen. The dog was mask-induced to anesthesia with isoflurane in oxygen, and anesthesia was maintained with isoflurane in oxygen and nitrous oxide. Fentanyl was administered for additional analgesia, and vecuronium bromide for muscle paralysis so as to facilitate retraction of the abdominal muscles and abdominal exploration. Exploration of the abdomen found that a Steinmann pin had caught the adventitia of the abdominal aorta approximately 1 cm cranial to the aortic bifurcation, and the aorta was wrapped around the pin, thus occluding aortic blood flow. Before cutting the pin and freeing the aorta, Rummel tourniquets were loosely placed around the aorta cranially and caudally to the obstruction. Shortly after freeing the aorta, blood flow returned to the hindquarters and bleeding occurred within the peritoneal cavity. The hemorrhage was stopped by occluding the aorta with the Rummel tourniquets. The source of hemorrhage was a tear in the vena cava, which was repaired with suture. After removing the Rummel tourniquets the other three pins were trimmed, the abdominal cavity was flushed with warm sterile saline (0.9% NaCl) solution, and the body wall was closed in a routine manner.

The dog's recovery was uneventful except for anemia that developed as a result of the hemorrhage and administration of fluids; the anemia was treated and corrected with a blood transfusion. Six days after surgery, with no complications other than the primary problem of hindquarter paralysis, the dog was discharged to its owners. The dog improved with time and was eventually able to walk although it had persistent sciatic nerve deficits.

Initial analysis of the case

The primary problem in this case, entrapment of the abdominal aorta by a Steinmann pin, was not due to anesthetic management. It was a surgical error, one that posed diagnostic challenges to the anesthetist because of what was initially perceived to be a monitor-related problem when in fact the problem was a patient-related one. Only after other information became available was it possible for the anesthetist and surgeon to identify and resolve the problem.

Investigation of the case

One of the issues in this case is how an anesthetist deals with a monitor—in this case a Doppler—that fails during anesthetic management of a patient. With regards to Doppler devices, they can and do fail for a variety of reasons, including loss of battery charge, electrical interference from other equipment, using an inadequate amount of conducting gel to maintain contact between probe and skin over an artery, or displacement of the probe when a patient moves or is being moved. Understandably, such failures, especially if they occur frequently, would lead an anesthetist to distrust these devices and would create a mindset—a rule—that when a Doppler stops working, it is most likely due to a problem with the Doppler rather than the patient; indeed, that was the initial mindset of the anesthetist of this case. But this mindset or bias, specifically ascertainment bias in which the anesthetist's thinking was shaped by prior experiences and expectations regarding the Doppler, and premature closure before verifying that indeed the Doppler had failed, shifted problem-solving efforts away from the patient to the monitoring device. The initial solution used in this particular case, that of getting another Doppler device and placing its probe over a forelimb artery, made it impossible to distinguish between a patient-related problem and a monitor-related problem.

A patient-oriented approach, one that would have made it possible to quickly distinguish between patient- and monitor-related problems, would have been to place the probe of the dubiously functioning Doppler over a forelimb artery. A blood-flow signal generated at the new location would have indicated that the problem was patient-related and not monitor-related. Alternatively, the anesthetist could have applied the probe to his own radial artery and quickly determined that the Doppler was working properly and that the loss of signal was patient-related. Another very simple, non-technical, patient-centered technique would have been to palpate arteries in the hindlimbs at the time the Doppler signal stopped and then palpate an artery in a forelimb; lack of a palpable pulse in a hindlimb artery and presence of one in a forelimb artery would have quickly identified the problem as patient-related.

In the day-to-day practice of anesthesia, monitoring devices fail and do so seemingly at the worst of times. When some monitoring devices fail they also sound their alarms, alarms that are meant to draw attention to patient-related problems. But the alarms, especially false alarms, can also be a source of distraction, irritation, and frustration for anesthetists. In a study of alarm occurrences, of 1455 alarm soundings, only eight represented critical and potentially life-threatening risk to the patients (Edworthy & Hellier 2006). Another study suggested that alarms indicated actual patient risk only 3% of the time they occurred, and were spurious in 75% of cases (Edworthy & Hellier 2006). Furthermore, alarms are often too loud and shrill. As a result they are irritating and can interfere with an anesthetist's performance. The overall result is that alarms are often turned off or disabled, thus defeating their purpose (Edworthy & Hellier 2006).

This case also demonstrates how easily an anesthetist's attention can be drawn away from the patient to a monitoring device. A reasonable question is, what process should the anesthetist have followed? A more appropriate question would be, what educational technique or approach should be used to train an anesthetist to first check the patient and then check the seemingly errant monitor? It is easy to tell someone that when a monitor sounds an alarm or malfunctions, he or she must first check the patient and then, once the patient's condition and wellbeing have been ascertained, turn to the monitor. But what assurance is there that this admonition will move from the person's short-term memory to long-term memory and result in a consistent pattern of behavior? An answer may be found in the neurobiology of learning.

Learning is optimized when a predictive stimulus or event and the event it predicts are very close in time. This is known as "temporal contiguity," which depends on learning a temporal map that is essential for association formation (Balsam & Gallistel 2009). This sounds rather esoteric and ivory tower, but an example may help to explain this concept.

Let's assume a goal of anesthesia training is that when a monitor alarm enunciates, the anesthetist, as a matter of routine, first checks the patient rather than checking the monitor or, worse yet, silences the alarm without checking the patient. In initial learning experiences, if the interval is very short between an alarm sounding (stimulus) and the trainee checking the patient (predicted and **desired** behavior), it is more likely that the trainee will encode the desired behavior, that is, on subsequent occasions will check the patient first and not the monitor and its alarm. This means that those involved in training residents, veterinary students, or technicians, must be close at hand so that when such an event occurs (an alarm sounds) the desired behavior can be impressed upon the trainee in a timely manner. In other words, the basis of skill acquisition is based on repetition of analytic processes until they become automatic (Stiegler & Tung 2014).

Another feature of this case, one that the anesthetist noticed and that was an important element in solving the dog's problem, was that after the first surgery the dog was not recovering as expected. This observation coupled with all of the other insights (Doppler device failure in the operating room, radiographic findings, lack of palpable pulses in the hindlimbs but palpable pulses in the forelimbs, and pale penile mucous membranes), led the anesthesia-surgical team to consider the Steinmann pins as a potential cause of the problem. This retrospective analysis and open, non-confrontational sharing of information by all team members during the dog's initial recovery, demonstrate the value of critically reviewing data collected during and after a problematic anesthetic episode. It is an example of effective communication. Such reviews (debriefings) help to identify problems that may not be obvious at a particular moment during a patient's anesthesia and have the advantage of drawing upon a number of individuals' perspectives of the case and increases the likelihood of identifying and solving problems.

Case 6.3

An owner brought his 5-day-old 68-kg thoroughbred foal to the large animal hospital because it had been straining to urinate since birth and had developed a distended abdomen over the previous 24 hours. At presentation the foal was bright and alert although it was tachycardic (144 beats per minute) and tachypneic (72 breaths per minute). Physical examination stressed the foal to such a degree that it became dyspneic and recumbent, both believed to be a result of respiratory difficulty due to its severe abdominal distension; its mucous membranes, which initially had been pink and moist, developed a bluish hue. Initial blood work was: hematocrit 33%, total plasma solids $7.0\,g\,dL^{-1}$, blood creatinine $380\,\mu mol\,L^{-1}$ (normal $<194\,\mu mol\,L^{-1}$). A sample of abdominal fluid had a creatinine concentration of $1724\,\mu mol\,L^{-1}$. The foal was hyperkalemic, hyponatremic, and hypochloremic. The presumptive diagnosis was a ruptured urinary bladder. After gaining the owner's informed consent, the foal was prepared for anesthesia and surgery, with anesthesia managed by the anesthesia resident on duty.

While the foal was awake, approximately 2–3 L of fluid was drained from the foal's abdomen, but further attempts to drain the abdomen were unsuccessful because the abdominal drain repeatedly became blocked. The foal was premedicated with midazolam and induced to anesthesia with fentanyl followed by ketamine, all given intravenously. The foal was intubated with a silicone 11-mm internal diameter endotracheal tube, which was then attached to the circle rebreathing circuit of a small animal anesthesia machine, started on isoflurane (3%) in oxygen ($2\,L\,min^{-1}$), and allowed to breathe spontaneously. While attaching the leads for the electrocardiogram and pulse oximeter the anesthetist noted that the breathing circuit's reservoir bag was moving in synchrony with the foal's breathing. A short time later when the foal was rolled into dorsal recumbency, its mucous membranes were noted to be gray and the pulse oximeter indicated an oxygen saturation of 52%. An attempt was made to give the foal a respiratory sigh by compressing the reservoir bag on the breathing circuit, but the bag was difficult to compress and resulted in very little if any movement of the foal's chest or abdomen.

At that moment another anesthetist entered the induction area to assist with case management. The anesthetist managing the patient stated that the foal could not be ventilated because of its fluid-distended abdomen. After a short discussion and inspection that included a quick palpation of the patient's abdomen, the second anesthetist commented that the difficulty of manually ventilating the foal (i.e., compressing the reservoir bag) seemed out of proportion to the degree of abdominal distention; indeed, the foal's abdomen was distended, but it was not "drum tight." While quickly inspecting the readily visible components of the breathing system, the second anesthetist noticed that the pilot balloon of the endotracheal tube cuff was overly distended. The cuff was deflated by removing approximately 20 mL of air from the cuff, after which the foal was easily ventilated. Within a few seconds of this maneuver, and despite delivering several breaths to the foal, it had a cardiac arrest. Cardiac resuscitation was successful, but the foal was euthanized the following day at the owner's request because of persistent central neurological deficits.

Analysis of the case

The most likely explanation as to why this foal was difficult to ventilate is that the cuff of the endotracheal tube was over-inflated and had herniated over the distal end of the tube thus obstructing the airway. Although an infrequent endotracheal tube-associated problem, it has been reported in humans (Szekely *et al.* 1993) and dogs (Bergadano *et al.* 2004). Over-inflation in and of itself is usually insufficient to cause an endotracheal tube cuff to herniate over the end of the tube; usually there is some other precipitating event such as a change in the position of the tube or patient. For example, during positioning of a patient, if a tube with an over-inflated cuff is accidentally pulled slightly out of the trachea, the cuff may adhere to the tracheal wall and then balloon over the distal end of the tube. Another factor favoring cuff herniation in this particular case and this particular endotracheal tube, is that the cuff material tends to become more pliable over time as it approaches the patient's body temperature; under the right conditions—overly inflated and moved—the warmed, pliable cuff can herniate over the distal end of the tube.

Another possible mechanism that could explain how the endotracheal tube became obstructed is that the over-inflated cuff compressed and collapsed the wall of the tube. This can happen in tubes that are old and have lost structural integrity. This endotracheal tube was not old and after the foal was extubated, inspection of the tube did not find evidence that it was structurally compromised.

One cannot exclude the possibility that the over-inflated cuff expanded eccentrically and forced the patient-end of the tube against the wall of the trachea, thus obstructing the airway. However, the tube used was a Murphy tube, one with a Murphy eye at its distal end, a feature that would have reduced the likelihood of airway obstruction by the tracheal wall and should have made ventilation easier than it was in this case.

The diagnosis of the problem occurred when the second anesthetist joined the case in progress in the induction room. During the hand-off of a patient from one caregiver to another, the caregiver who is taking over the patient has a fresh perspective of the case, a situation that increases the likelihood of detecting errors, such as fixation errors (De Keyser & Woods 1990; Guerlain et al. 1999). In this particular case a hand-off was not occurring, but the second anesthetist gained another perspective of the situation, what some would describe as bringing "fresh eyes" to the problem (Reason 1990; Webster 2005). Indeed, the error literature is replete with many examples in which accidents were avoided or quickly resolved by the timely intervention of individuals who were naive to the error in progress and thus not biased as to the nature of the problem. A learning issue in this case is that it is always appropriate to ask for help or seek a second opinion when managing a difficult patient, or when the case is not progressing as planned or intended. It is counterproductive to remain stuck in a problem-solving loop that fails to move problem-solving from the skill-based and rule-based levels to the next higher level, that of knowledge-based problem-solving, which requires the effortful analytical mode of cognition (Figure 6.5). Often it takes "fresh eyes" to break out of the loop to see the larger picture and solve the problem.

Investigation of the case

The initial error that caused this incident was over-inflation of the cuff and its herniation over the end of the endotracheal tube. But why and how was it inflated too much? To answer that question we need to look at the environment—the system—in which the error occurred. In this particular hospital, 60-mL syringes were routinely used to inflate the cuffs of large animal endotracheal tubes; these syringes were readily kept at hand in the induction rooms and surgical suites, usually on the anesthesia machines or anesthesia supply carts. This meant that as a matter of routine, regardless of the size of either the patient or endotracheal tube used, one of these 60-mL syringes was readily available and routinely used to inflate endotracheal tube cuffs.

In this particular case the endotracheal tube had an internal diameter of 11 mm and a low-volume, high-pressure cuff, one that typically requires only about 10 mL of air to be fully inflated; volumes of air above 10 mL are excessive. By using a 60-mL syringe whoever inflated the cuff was likely to exceed the maximum volume needed to safely inflate it. In fact a person's tendency when pulling on the plunger to fill this size of syringe with air, is to withdraw the syringe plunger at least halfway (~30 mL) and in most cases past the 45-mL mark (J.W.L., unpublished observations). In addition, there was no mechanism in place to prevent the anesthetist from using the large-volume syringe on a small-volume cuff, nor was there a forcing mechanism associated with the syringe that would limit the volume of air that could be drawn into it.

A strategy the anesthetist could have used to avoid over-inflating the cuff would have been to compress the reservoir bag on the breathing circuit while the cuff was being inflated. While listening to the sound of air escaping around the endotracheal tube the anesthetist could have continued to inflate the cuff until it just stopped the leak of gas around the tube at an airway pressure no greater that 20 cmH$_2$O. Using this technique the cuff would have been sufficiently inflated to prevent the leak of airway gas up to an airway pressure of 20 cmH$_2$O, but would have allowed a leak at or above that limit. This maneuver lessens the likelihood of over-inflating the cuff and reduces the risk of producing a high contact pressure between the endotracheal tube cuff and tracheal mucosa, thus preserving capillary blood flow in the tracheal mucosa. For whatever reason this technique was not used. Since the case did not undergo post hoc analysis it is impossible to know what the conditions were at the time that led to omission of this technique for inflating endotracheal tube cuffs.

A number of other causal factors were involved in this case. The resident was in training, a fact suggesting that the training program had failed to adequately teach the resident how to work through problems when schemata and rule-based solutions fail. In this case the resident's decision-making processes seemed to involve at least three types of cognitive errors: coning of attention, fixation bias, and confirmation bias. Possibly under the stress of the situation the resident concentrated on one piece of information to the exclusion of other information that was relevant to the problem at hand.

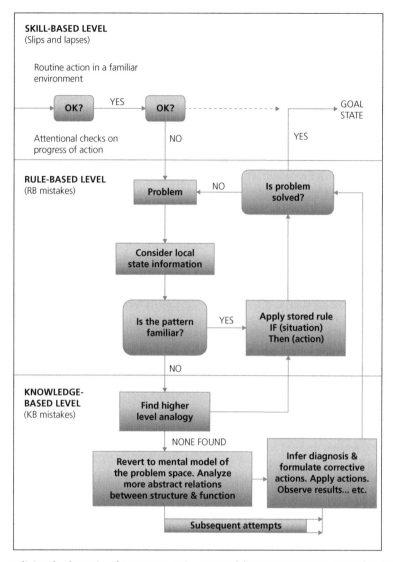

Figure 6.5 Schematic outlining the dynamics of Reason's generic error modeling system (GEMS). Central to this model is that humans are strongly biased to search for and find a pre-packaged solution to a problem at the Rule-Based Level. Only after cycling around this rule-based route and not finding a satisfactory solution will people resort to the far more effortful Knowledge-Based Level of problem-solving even when circumstances demand this approach at the outset. From: Reason, J.T. (1990) *Human Error*. Cambridge, UK: Cambridge University Press, p. 64. With permission of the publisher.

The resident also sought evidence supporting the earlier working hypothesis (i.e., that the abdomen was distended to the point of causing respiratory distress) while ignoring information that contradicted it (e.g., when physically palpated, the abdomen actually was not overly distended). The training program should have taught the resident to systematically work through any problem by following a step-wise process that would include checking the patency of the endotracheal tube. This process would include deflating and reinflating the cuff, even potentially extubating and reintubating the patient, procedures that would have identified the problem. The latter step, that of extubating and reintubating a patient, is never undertaken lightly for fear of not being able to reintubate the patient. However, by taking this step, the anesthetist's attention would have been drawn to the over-inflated pilot balloon, which would have triggered the realization that there was an airway issue, not an issue of a distended abdomen compressing the thoracic cavity. Being able to work through the diagnostic process involves education, training, and experience.

Education strategies directed at improving formal and experiential knowledge, are crucial in error prevention (Monteiro *et al.* 2015). Having knowledge of possible airway complications, how they can occur, and knowing how to manage them, should be an important element of any anesthesia training program. After all, few complications can kill a patient faster than a "failed airway." Indeed, the single largest category of anesthetic-related injury in human patients is respiratory events, and the three main causes of respiratory-related injury are inadequate ventilation, esophageal intubation, and difficult tracheal intubation (Engel *et al.* 2004). Of the three, difficult tracheal intubation accounts for 17% of the respiratory-related injuries and results in significant morbidity and mortality; up to 28% of all human deaths associated with anesthesia are due to the inability to mask-ventilate or intubate the patient (Engel *et al.* 2004). In a study by Cooper *et al.* (2002), most of the preventable incidents involved human error (82%).

Do these incidents occur frequently in veterinary anesthesia? The answer is unknown. However, there are a number of reports describing a variety of airway complications following intubation of horses (Abrahamsen *et al.* 1990; Heath *et al.* 1989; Holland *et al.* 1986; Touzot-Jourde *et al.* 2005; Trim 1984). It has been suggested that inadequate monitoring and unrecognized or untreated respiratory depression are the most common causes of anesthetic death in veterinary

medicine (Alef & Oechtering 1998). The fact that anesthesia-associated morbidity and mortality are higher in veterinary anesthesia than in human anesthesia suggests that airway-associated incidents likely do occur in veterinary anesthesia; this case adds credence to that contention. Training anesthetists to recognize and manage these complications when they occur should be an important part of an anesthesia training program.

The most reliable method for determining that an endotracheal tube has been properly inserted into the trachea is to directly visualize the tube passing between the arytenoids; this is primary, clinical-based evidence. When direct vision is not possible, the usual situation when anesthetizing large animals such as horses and cattle, tube position must be confirmed by using other techniques or equipment (secondary or technologic evidence) that provide reliable evidence that the trachea has been intubated; examples include:

- **End-tidal CO_2 detector**—only confirms the presence of CO_2, which suggests that the endotracheal tube is somewhere in the airway, which includes the mouth, nose, pharynx, and larynx. Carbon dioxide in the stomach from any source is less prominent than respiratory CO_2 and tends to diminish with each breath when the esophagus has been intubated accidentally.
- **Esophageal detectors: self-inflating bulb or airway syringe**—will distinguish between esophageal and tracheal intubation (Figure 6.6). For the flexible bulb the user compresses it and attaches it to the machine-end of the endotracheal tube, or, if using the syringe, pulls back the plunger of the syringe that is attached to the endotracheal tube. Both devices create a vacuum in the endotracheal tube. If the tube is

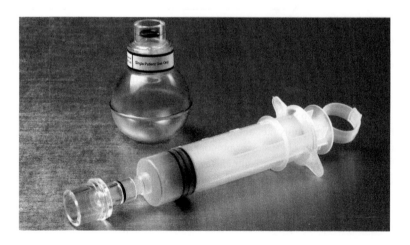

Figure 6.6 Esophageal detectors, such as this bulb and syringe, can be used to determine if an endotracheal tube has been inserted into the trachea or the esophagus of an anesthetized small animal patient. With permission of the manufacturer, CareStream Medical Ltd; Coquitlam, British Columbia, Canada.

in the esophagus, the vacuum will pull the esophageal mucosa against the distal end of the endotracheal tube and prevent the bulb from re-expanding, or prevent the syringe's plunger from being withdrawn (Rudraraju & Eisen 2009). In veterinary medicine these detectors can only be used in patients intubated with endotracheal tubes that have standard 15-mm connectors, a fact that precludes their use in most large animal patients; in this particular case, since the foal was intubated with an endotracheal tube that had a 15-mm connector, either of these esophageal detectors could have been used. Use of an esophageal detector is recommended in patients with cardiac arrest because exhaled CO_2 in these patients is normally low and a CO_2 gas monitor will reflect low pulmonary blood flow rather than failed intubation (Anonymous 2000; Rudraraju & Eisen 2009).

Of the first two methods listed above, the Advanced Cardiovascular Life Support (ACLS) recommendations state that airway CO_2 monitors are rated good to very good for discriminating between tracheal or esophageal intubation, and esophageal detectors are rated fair to good (Anonymous 2000; Rudraraju & Eisen 2009). Other methods are less reliable, but include:

- **Auscultation of the thorax**—At least in human patients, this method has been found to be a less reliable method because of noisy environments or referred sounds, especially in the presence of pulmonary disease.
- **Palpation**—palpating the neck around the trachea to check if there are "two tracheas." This is possible in some animals, but anatomy or body form/condition of a patient may render this impractical in others, such as an anesthetized pig, or a very obese animal, or an animal with extensive neck injuries.
- **Condensation**—condensation inside the tube is not always reliable because warm, moist gas from the stomach can cause fogging of the endotracheal tube.
- **Movement of the reservoir bag**—when properly intubated, the reservoir bag will move in synchrony with the patient's respirations, i.e., during inspiration the reservoir bag will diminish in size and during exhalation it will expand. However, when the esophagus is intubated the reservoir bag may still move in synchrony with ventilation, but will do so paradoxically, i.e., as the patient inhales, the reservoir bag will increase in size, and during exhalation it will decrease in size. These paradoxical movements occur because gas in the stomach and esophagus undergoes changes

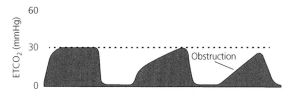

Figure 6.7 Capnogram showing airway obstruction due to kinking of an endotracheal tube. Adapted from a graphic developed by Welch Allyn. Permission granted by Welch Allyn.

in volume due to respiratory-induced changes in airway pressure; the resulting compression and expansion of esophageal and gastric gases are transmitted to the reservoir bag, which will move as the patient breathes, but do so paradoxically. This phenomenon is more likely to occur when there is a significant amount of gas in the esophagus or stomach.

In other words, there are a number of strategies that an anesthetist can and must use to confirm that a patient has been correctly intubated.

The most typical signs that an endotracheal tube is obstructed are decreased thoracic excursions and tidal volume, absence of gas flow through the endotracheal tube, change in the morphology of the capnogram waveform (Figure 6.7), and increased airway pressures during the inspiratory phase of assisted or controlled ventilation (Bergadano *et al.* 2004). Changes in patient oxygenation can be only late indicators of a problem; in a report involving two dogs, hemoglobin desaturation (SpO_2) occurred between 6 and 8 minutes after cuff herniation (Bergadano *et al.* 2004).

Identifying the 60-mL syringe as a key element in this error seems overly simplistic at best. Could it really be a key latent condition that contributed to this error? This question may be best answered with another question: "What would have happened if there had only been a 10-mL syringe available for inflating the endotracheal tube cuff?" Indeed, it can be the small details that set the stage for errors.

Case 6.4

It was late March in an upper Midwestern state and an Alaskan malamute was scheduled for anesthesia and surgical correction of keratoconjunctivitis sicca by transposition of its parotid duct to the affected eye. The dog was 5 years old, weighed 75 kg, and was slightly overweight (3/5 body score). The owners stated that the dog was in good health and a physical examination and quick assessment tests (hematocrit, total plasma solids, blood urea nitrogen, and blood glucose) confirmed their assessment. The dog was noted to have its dense winter fur coat, but this was expected as it had been a long, cold winter.

For anesthesia the dog was premedicated with acepromazine, oxymorphone, and glycopyrrolate, all combined in one syringe and given IM. After 25 minutes the dog was induced to anesthesia with ketamine and diazepam, intubated, and attached to a circle system to which isoflurane in oxygen was delivered while the dog breathed spontaneously. After surgical preparation the dog was moved to the operating room where it was placed in dorsal recumbency on the surgery table, and cloth restraints were used to gently pull its forelimbs caudally away from the head. A circulating warm water pad was placed under the dog to help maintain body temperature during surgery. The dog was instrumented for monitoring of electrocardiogram, capnometry ($P_E'CO_2$), pulse oximetry (SpO_2), and indirect blood pressure before it was covered with surgical drapes. The isoflurane vaporizer setting, which had been at 1.5%, was turned down to 1.0%.

After approximately one hour of surgery the anesthetist commented that the dog seemed light because the heart rate had increased from 95 beats per minute to 130 beats per minute, mean arterial blood pressure had increased from 75 mmHg to 87 mmHg, and respiratory rate had increased from 10 breaths/min to 17; the anesthetist turned the vaporizer dial setting from 1.0% to 1.75%. At this time the SpO_2 was 95% and $P_E'CO_2$ 35 mmHg, having decreased from 47 mmHg. The eye reflexes (palpebral response or nystagmus) and position were unavailable for assessment and the surgeon did not comment on their presence or absence.

Half an hour later the dog appeared to be very light despite the vaporizer dial setting having been increased to 2.5%. The heart rate was 147 beats per minute, mean blood pressure was 95 mmHg, and respiratory rate was 23 breaths per minute; the anesthetist also mentioned that the dog seemed to be moving. The SpO_2 was 96% and $P_E'CO_2$ 33 mmHg. Additional oxymorphone and acepromazine were given intravenously, and the vaporizer dial was turned down to 2.0%. The dog seemed to settle down for about 10 minutes after which the monitored variables began to increase yet again. During this time the vaporizer dial setting had been left unchanged at 2.0%.

The anesthetist solicited a second opinion about patient management. While talking with the anesthetist, the consulting anesthetist palpated the dog's paws and commented that they felt quite warm. A thermometer indicated a rectal temperature of 40.8 °C. The circulating warm water pad was promptly removed from under the dog, the surgical drapes were removed without interfering with the surgical field, and the dog's inguinal area was lightly bathed with alcohol. The vaporizer dial was turned to 1.0%, remained there for approximately 10 minutes, and then was turned to 0.7% where it remained until the end of surgery.

Initial analysis of the case

In this patient the hyperthermia produced some confusing signs—tachycardia, hypertension, hyperventilation, and even the appearance of movement. These signs led the anesthetist to believe the dog was "light" and responding to surgical stimulation, an assessment that prompted the anesthetist to increase the vaporizer dial setting and administer intravenously two drugs for additional analgesia and tranquilization. Once the hyperthermia was diagnosed it became obvious that the signs were a mix of confusing signals. Indeed, in anesthetized dogs as body temperature increases from normal up to 42 °C, more inhalant anesthetic is needed (Steffey & Eger 1974). However, if more anesthetic is administered, either by increasing the vaporizer dial setting or by administering injectable anesthetics, or both, and the dog continues to appear to be light, one must suspect that something else is amiss with the patient.

It could be said this case is nothing more than an example of what happens when an anesthetized dog becomes hyperthermic, one that describes an appropriate strategy for treating that condition. But it is more than this. It is an example of a near miss—if hyperthermia had continued to be unrecognized and untreated it could have progressed and triggered a cascade of undesirable effects, such as CNS dysfunction (Steffey & Eger 1974), and become an adverse incident. The dog also received drugs that did nothing for the hyperthermia and, once the hyperthermia was diagnosed and treated, resulted in a relative overdose of inhalant anesthetic. This is an example of a rule-based error in which a good rule (**if** an anesthetized animal is too light, **then** deepen the plane of anesthesia) is misapplied because the dog's underlying condition was not diagnosed. The anesthetist seemingly remained fixated on the belief that the physiological signs were due to surgical stimulation even though the dog did not respond as expected to additional drugs and its plane of anesthesia remained light. Much to the anesthetist's credit, and what helped move decision-making to the knowledge-based analytical mode of thinking, was the request for assistance with patient management. This resulted in identification and resolution of the problem.

Investigation of the case

Monitoring involves the regular and periodic assessment of many patient-related variables and their parameters so as to determine the patient's depth of anesthesia and its response to both anesthesia and the procedure it is undergoing (see Appendix C "ACVAA Monitoring Guidelines," and Appendix D "ACVAA Guidelines for Anesthesia of Horses"). In this particular case the anesthetist did monitor the patient with the focus primarily on the cardiopulmonary system. Other variables that would have provided more insight as to the patient's condition, such as body temperature, muscle tone, movement, and eye signs, were either not monitored or incorrectly interpreted. So how could the anesthetist break out of cycling around the rule-based loop that is a prominent feature of Reason's General Errors Model, and move to the analytical mode of problem-solving? One strategy would be to use mnemonics, such as 3-P (see "Mnemonics" in Chapter 8), which are meant to help anesthetists re-evaluate clinical situations when they are not going as expected or desired, and prompt them to use the analytical mode of thinking (Stiegler & Ruskin 2012). In this case, after the first administration of oxymorphone and acepromazine failed to deepen the plane of anesthesia, the anesthetist needed to re-evaluate the assumption that the patient's only problem was that it was too light and reacting to surgical stimulation; the patient's condition needed to be more fully assessed, as the 3-P mnemonic suggests.

In essence this near miss shows how signs during anesthesia can be confusing when one has to distinguish between physiological responses to increased surgical stimulation (nociception) and those due to other causes such as hyperthermia. The first situation is common, one that all anesthetists can relate to. In fact it may be one of the most common complications requiring intervention in anesthesia. Arousal or breakthrough pain requiring the unplanned administration of

a dose of intravenous anesthetic or analgesic, was reported in almost 15% of 1386 small animal anesthetics, almost 22% of which involved anesthetized dogs (McMillan & Darcy 2016). So it is not surprising that this was the first complication that came to the anesthetist's mind; a classic "flesh and blood" diagnosis. In fact, it is perhaps so common that most anesthetists do not consider it a complication at all, but think of it as a typical event requiring a standard response during anesthesia and surgery.

Unlike hypothermia, hyperthermia is not a common complication, so it is not surprising that it was not the first complication the anesthetist considered. In retrospect, given the dog's breed (hairy, large breed dog), hyperthermia should have been on the anesthetist's list of probable complications. However, even without anticipating this complication, the anesthetist should have considered the signs as not specific to surgical stimulation, but as a typical general response to any physiological stressor, any one of which can be life threatening. For example, hypoxemia ($P_aO_2 < 60\,mmHg$) or hypercarbemia ($P_aCO_2 > 50\,mmHg$) can also cause an increase in sympathetic nervous system activity that increases heart and respiratory rates, and blood pressure. So once the anesthetist had attempted and seemingly failed to correct the patient's condition—patient is "light" and responding to surgical manipulation—a thorough check of the patient and monitors would have been appropriate so as to identify other patient-associated problems. By doing so the anesthetist would have rapidly identified the hyperthermia. Mnemonics such as those discussed in Chapter 8 (see "COVER ABCD and A SWIFT CHECK" in Chapter 8), would help rule in or rule out the common causes of complications encountered during anesthesia. Using such techniques in this case could have assisted analytical problem-solving and would have ensured that body temperature was assessed.

Near miss vignettes

Vignette 6.1

A dog scheduled for an endoscopic examination was sedated, catheterized intravenously, and induced to anesthesia in one room and then, once it was determined to be stable, transported on a cart to the endoscopy exam room. Once in the endoscopy suite the usual routine was to start the flow of oxygen from the anesthesia machine, attach the patient to the machine's breathing circuit, turn on the vaporizer, check the patient to make sure its heart was beating and the patient was breathing, and then attach monitoring devices such as pulse oximeter, electrocardiogram leads, and blood pressure cuff. However, on this particular occasion, as the anesthesia technician and the patient entered the endoscopy suite, the endoscopist and medicine resident promptly began positioning and preparing the dog for endoscopy. This made it difficult for the anesthesia technician to work around the patient and connect it to the anesthesia circuit and attach monitoring devices. Within a few minutes the patient seemed appropriately positioned for endoscopy and instrumented for monitoring. At this time another anesthetist entered the room to see if the first anesthetist needed assistance and noticed that the oxygen flow meter was not turned on. This omission was quickly corrected.

This incident demonstrates how omissions can occur—in this case a capture slip that resulted in omitting to turn on the oxygen. The anesthesia technician felt pressured by the endoscopist to prepare the dog for endoscopy before it was fully instrumented and its anesthesia stabilized. In addition, the role of hierarchy probably made the technician feel pressured. The technician's routine for managing these types of patients was interrupted and in the press of the moment and the distractions of working around the endoscopist and resident, the technician forgot to turn on the oxygen. To help prevent this in the future the anesthesia technician was assured that in this type of situation any anesthetist had every right to request the endoscopist, or any doctor, to wait until the anesthetized patient was appropriately and safely anesthetized and monitored. This incident was described during the section's weekly rounds so as to show how errors can occur, and to help convey the message that it is OK to tell a doctor to wait until the anesthetist has stabilized the patient for the procedure.

Vignette 6.2

A dog that had been hit by a car had its fractured tibia repaired under general inhalant anesthesia. The animal was instrumented for monitoring blood pressure, pulse oximetry, airway gases, and body temperature. Anesthesia and surgery, performed late in the evening, proceeded uneventfully. Post-op radiographs were necessary and the dog was prepared for transport to the radiology suite. The anesthetist decided to transport the dog on a gurney without a vaporizer or circle system and did so in the belief that time would be saved by not having to deal with the operational details of the cart-mounted anesthesia machine. It was also assumed that the patent was sufficiently oxygenated so that the short trip to radiology would not adversely affect oxygenation. The patient was quickly transported to radiology where it was discovered that the radiology suite was locked and the person on duty was not in the area. The animal was promptly wheeled to the anesthesia induction area and attached to an anesthesia machine. The person covering radiology eventually returned, the dog was moved back to radiology, all procedures were completed without further incident, and the dog recovered uneventfully from anesthesia.

This particular case of a near miss highlights not only how assumptions can lead to errors in decision-making, but upon closer inspection identifies many unforeseen factors that could have, under the right circumstances, led to an adverse incident. In this case there were several errors in decision-making: the assumption that transporting the patient to radiology would proceed quickly and uneventfully; an assumption that the radiology area was prepared for the patient; and a failure to communicate the intended plan to the radiology person on duty. As discussed in Chapter 2 (see "Error causation: organizational and supervision factors" and "Individual responsibility within an organization"), a hallmark of high reliability organizations and the attitudes of people who work within such organizations, is a preoccupation with failure and the assumption that each day will be a bad day, so the people behave accordingly (Weick 2002). Communication is crucial in preventing errors; inadequate communication, such as occurred in this case, is cited as one of the most common causes of preventable errors (Brindley 2014). But closer inspection of this case reveals other "traps" that although present, fortunately did not come to the fore and cause patient harm.

In this scenario, moving the anesthetized patient from the operating room to the radiology suite required moving the patient from the surgical table to a cart while maintaining anesthesia and transferring all the accoutrements necessary to maintain anesthesia, such as intravenous catheters, endotracheal tube, intravenous fluids if still being administered, pumps if being used, and monitoring equipment. The complexity and hazards of patient transport have been described in veterinary anesthesia (Kennedy & Smith 2014). During transport, care must be taken to prevent physical harm to the patient, such as can occur if an appendage is dangling off the side of the transport cart as it is pushed through doorways, preventing a doorknob or handle from snagging an intravenous line, or catching a breathing circuit hose and extubating the patient; the list of hazards (latent conditions) is endless. In this case none of these latent conditions triggered an incident, but they were present and had something happened to trigger one, then the optimistic assumptions about the safety of the transport process would have been rendered moot.

During case management it is not unusual to take shortcuts and there can be many reasons for doing so, such as an attempt to improve efficiency. Indeed, shortcuts can be a sign of inefficient standard operating procedures that, although well intentioned, actually make a task or job more difficult to perform or time consuming. But shortcuts may bypass cuing mechanisms that are normally present when standard procedures are followed; their absence can lead to slips, lapses, and errors of omission. During patient transport there are often interruptions and distractions that can lead to capture slips and omissions, which could lead to patient harm. In this case the locked and unattended radiology area was an interruption in the patient transport process that caused the error to become manifest, that is, the action did not go as planned and placed the patient at risk of harm.

Patients under general inhalant anesthesia are usually well saturated with oxygen, as indicated by partial pressures of oxygen often above 400 mmHg. One could assume that an anesthetized patient could be disconnected from one anesthesia machine, transported a short distance, and attached to another anesthesia machine without a significant or dangerous decrease in oxygen saturation. Again, this assumes that nothing will interfere with the transport process, that there will be no delays due to latent conditions waiting to be activated by the right circumstances.

Conclusion

The errors in clinical reasoning and decision-making highlighted in this chapter were unintentionally made by intelligent, caring people. As stated previously, when

reading these cases and near miss vignettes, it is difficult to understand why those involved, be they single individuals or teams, missed or could not see what is so obvious to us in the here and now. And it is this very aspect of how errors occur that makes learning from them so difficult: we were not there when the errors occurred and really do not understand the many conditions and factors at play at the time and place—the context—in which they occurred. But this is exactly what we must do to understand how errors evolve. We need to dig deep to find the root causes of the error or get as close to them as we can; only then do we have a chance of preventing future errors.

References

Abrahamsen, E.J., *et al.* (1990) Bilateral arytenoid cartilage paralysis after inhalation anesthesia in a horse. *Journal of the American Veterinary Medical Association* **197**(10): 1363–1365.

Alef, M. & Oechtering, G. (1998) [Reflections on anesthetic risk]. *Tierärztliche Praxis Ausgabe Kleintiere Heimtiere* **26**(5): 302–314.

Anonymous (2000) Part 6: Advanced cardiovascular life support: Section 3: Adjuncts for oxygenation, ventilation, and airway control. *Circulation* **102**(Suppl. 1): 95–104.

Balla, J., *et al.* (2012) Identifying early warning signs for diagnostic errors in primary care: A qualitative study. *BMJ Open* **2**(5); doi:10.1136/bmjopen-2012-001539.

Balsam, P.D. & Gallistel, C.R. (2009) Temporal maps and informativeness in associative learning. *Trends in Neurosciences* **32**(2): 73–78.

Bergadano, A., *et al.* (2004) Two cases of intraoperative herniation of the endotracheal tube cuff. *Schweizer Archiv für Tierheilkunde* **146**(12): 565–569.

Brindley, P.G. (2014) I. improving teamwork in anaesthesia and critical care: Many lessons still to learn. *British Journal of Anaesthesia* **112**(3): 399–401.

Cooper, J.B., *et al.* (2002) Preventable anesthesia mishaps: A study of human factors. *Quality and Safety in Health Care* **11**(3): 277–282.

Croskerry, P. (2003) The importance of cognitive errors in diagnosis and strategies to minimize them. *Academic Medicine: Journal of the Association of American Medical Colleges* **78**(8): 775–780.

Croskerry, P. (2005) Diagnostic failure: a cognitive and affective approach. In: *Advances in Patient Safety: From Research to Implementation (Volume 2: Concepts and Methodology)* (eds K. Henriksen, J.B. Battles, E.S. Marks & D.I. Lewin). Rockville, MD: Agency for Healthcare Research and Quality, pp. 241–254.

Croskerry, P. (2013) From mindless to mindful practice — cognitive bias and clinical decision making. *New England Journal of Medicine* **368**(26): 2445–2448.

De Keyser, V. & Woods, D.D. (1990) Fixation errors: failures to revise situation assessment in dynamic and risky systems. In: *Systems Reliability Assessment* (eds A.G. Colombo & A. Saiz de Bustamante). Kluwer Academic, pp. 231–251.

Edworthy, J. & Hellier, E. (2006) Alarms and human behaviour: Implications for medical alarms. *British Journal of Anaesthesia* **97**(1): 12–17.

Engel, T.P., Applegate, R.L., Chung, D.M., & Sanchez, A. (2004) *Management of the Difficult Airway*, Second; Version 1.0 edn. Global Anesthesiology Network (GASNet).

Graber, M.L., *et al.* (2005) Diagnostic error in internal medicine. *Archives of Internal Medicine* **165**(13): 1493–1499.

Graber, M.L. (2013) The incidence of diagnostic error in medicine. *BMJ Quality & Safety* **22**(Suppl. 2); ii21–ii27.

Guerlain, S.A., *et al.* (1999) Interactive critiquing as a form of decision support: An empirical evaluation. *Human Factors* **41**(1): 72–89.

Heath, R.B., *et al.* (1989) Laryngotracheal lesions following routine orotracheal intubation in the horse. *Equine Veterinary Journal* **21**(6): 434–437.

Holland, M., *et al.* (1986) Laryngotracheal injury associated with nasotracheal intubation in the horse. *Journal of the American Veterinary Medical Association* **189**(11): 1447–1450.

Kennedy, M.J. & Smith, L.J. (2014) Anesthesia case of the month. Accidental lidocaine overdose during surgery for vertebral fractures. *Journal of the American Veterinary Medical Association* **245**(10): 1098–1101.

McMillan, M. & Darcy, H. (2016) Adverse event surveillance in small animal anaesthesia: An intervention-based, voluntary reporting audit. *Veterinary Anaesthesia and Analgesia* **43**(2): 128–135.

Monteiro, S.D., *et al.* (2015) Reflecting on diagnostic errors: Taking a second look is not enough. *Journal of General Internal Medicine* **30**(9): 1270–1274.

Norman, G.R. & Eva, K.W. (2010) Diagnostic error and clinical reasoning. *Medical Education* **44**(1): 94–100.

Oxtoby, C., *et al.* (2015) We need to talk about error: Causes and types of error in veterinary practice. *Veterinary Record* **177**(17): 438–445.

Reason, J.T. (1990) *Human Error*. Cambridge: Cambridge University Press.

Reason, J.T. (2004) Beyond the organisational accident: The need for "error wisdom" on the frontline. *Quality and Safety in Health Care* **13**(Suppl. 2): ii28–ii33.

Rudraraju, P. & Eisen, L.A. (2009) Confirmation of endotracheal tube position: A narrative review. *Journal of Intensive Care Medicine* **24**(5): 283–292.

Steffey, E.P. & Eger, E.I. (1974) Hyperthermia and halothane MAC in the dog. *Anesthesiology* **41**(4): 392–396.

Stiegler, M.P., *et al.* (2012) Cognitive errors detected in anaesthesiology: A literature review and pilot study. *British Journal of Anaesthesia* **108**(2): 229–235.

Stiegler, M.P. & Ruskin, K.J. (2012) Decision-making and safety in anesthesiology. *Current Opinion in Anaesthesiology* **25**(6): 724–729.

Stiegler, M.P. & Tung, A. (2014) Cognitive processes in anesthesiology decision making. *Anesthesiology* **120**(1): 204–217.

Szekely, S.M., *et al.* (1993) The Australian Incident Monitoring Study. Problems related to the endotracheal tube: An analysis of 2000 incident reports. *Anaesthesia and Intensive Care* **21**(5): 611–616.

Touzot-Jourde, G., *et al.* (2005) The effects of two endotracheal tube cuff inflation pressures on liquid aspiration and tracheal wall damage in horses. *Veterinary Anaesthesia and Analgesia* **32**(1): 23–29.

Trim, C.M. (1984) Complications associated with the use of the cuffless endotracheal tube in the horse. *Journal of the American Veterinary Medical Association* **185**(5): 541–542.

Webster, C.S. (2005) The nuclear power industry as an alternative analogy for safety in anaesthesia and a novel approach for the conceptualisation of safety goals. *Anaesthesia* **60**(11): 1115–1122.

Weick, K.E. (2002) The reduction of medical errors through mindful interdependence. In: *Medical Errors: What Do We Know? What Do We Do?* (eds M.M. Rosenthal & K.M. Sutcliffe), 1st edn. San Francisco, CA: Jossey-Bass, pp. 177–199.

CHAPTER 7

Errors of Communication and Teamwork in Veterinary Anesthesia

> …larger improvements in seeing should occur when people with more diverse skills, experience, and perspectives think together in a context of respectful interaction.
>
> *Karl E. Weick (2002)*

It has become increasingly obvious that factors such as communication, teamwork, and leadership have significant roles in patient safety (Nagpal *et al.* 2012). Of these factors, communication is perhaps the most significant, both as a skill in itself and because effective communication is integral to the success of all other parts of the "system" (Nagpal *et al.* 2012). It's the glue that binds. Indeed, it is the critical factor if healthcare teams are to deliver effective and safe care to patients.

As discussed previously (see "Communication: what it is and how it fails" in Chapter 2), communication is the process by which information is passed orally or in written form from one individual to another. But communications can break down and do so in three ways: (1) information is never communicated because it is missing or incomplete; (2) during the communication process information is misunderstood or transmitted poorly (a poor method or structure is used for communication); and (3) once communicated the information is forgotten, inaccurately received, or interpreted incorrectly. In healthcare, when communication breaks down patient safety is jeopardized, a reality that has been documented in a number of clinical settings, including general medicine, emergency departments, and surgery (Brindley 2014; Greenberg *et al.* 2007; Lingard *et al.* 2004).

Teamwork is the array of interconnected behaviors, cognitive processes, and attitudes that make coordinated and adaptive performance possible in complex environments such as clinical settings (Salas *et al.* 2008). Not surprisingly when communication breakdowns occur teamwork is less than optimal and patient safety is jeopardized (Brindley 2014; Lingard *et al.* 2004). Based on evidence from acute care medicine it has been claimed that inadequate teamwork (and the related topic of inadequate communication) is one of our most common reasons for preventable error (Brindley 2014). A recent set of proposals for improving diagnosis in healthcare included the facilitation of teamwork as one of eight major goals (Bunting & Groszkruger 2016).

Is communication an issue in veterinary medicine? We would be naive to think otherwise. Indeed, recent reports confirm that communication breakdowns do contribute to errors in veterinary medicine (Kinnison *et al.* 2015; Oxtoby *et al.* 2015). The following cases and near miss vignette are examples of breakdowns in communication within the context of veterinary anesthesia.

Cases

Case 7.1

A 1-year-old, 18.2-kg hound-cross bitch was brought into the emergency receiving service of a referral practice. The owner's primary concern was that the dog was pregnant and had been straining to deliver puppies over the past 48 hours. When asked about the breeding date the owner stated the dog ran free but the owner had observed her being bred approximately 2 months previously by a local dog. The only other item in the dog's history was that she had been hit by a car 5 months previously but without any lasting effects. The emergency service clinician on duty was a surgeon who promptly

Errors in Veterinary Anesthesia, First Edition. John W. Ludders and Matthew McMillan.
© 2017 John Wiley & Sons, Inc. Published 2017 by John Wiley & Sons, Inc.

took the dog to radiology for an abdominal ultrasound examination that was performed by a visiting veterinary radiologist. The ultrasound exam was difficult as the bitch was uncooperative; the ultrasound was interpreted as indicating that there was one fetus. The dog was taken to the anesthesia section for induction of anesthesia and an emergency caesarean section.

When presenting the dog to the anesthesia service, the surgeon demanded that the patient be anesthetized immediately so that the puppy could be saved. The anesthetist on duty asked for more information about the patient, but was told in an abrupt manner to "quit delaying and get the dog on the table." Undeterred by this admonition, the anesthetist proceeded to perform a quick physical examination. The dog was found to be unkempt and nervous. She became aggressive when abdominal palpation was attempted and had to be muzzled. Her heart rate was 138 beats per minute and she was panting. Mucous membranes were pink and capillary refill time was 2 seconds. Her temperature was 39.9 °C, hematocrit was 31%, total plasma solids were 5.8 g dL^{-1}, blood urea nitrogen (Azostix) 1.8–5.4 mmol L^{-1}, and blood glucose 3.83 mmol L^{-1}.

Under the assumption that the bitch was pregnant and so as not to depress the fetus any more than necessary, she was not premedicated. A catheter was inserted into a cephalic vein, she was administered oxygen by mask for 5 minutes, and then induced to anesthesia with propofol. The dog's trachea was intubated and the endotracheal tube was connected to a circle circuit delivering isoflurane (1%) in oxygen (2 L min^{-1}). When positioned in dorsal recumbency the vaporizer was increased to 2% because the dog seemed light. It was also noted that her thorax had poor compliance as it was difficult to manually ventilate her and the thoracic wall did not move to the extent expected for the size of the manually delivered tidal volumes. The position of the endotracheal tube was reassessed and because of remaining doubts as to the position of the endotracheal tube, the dog was extubated and reintubated. Despite this maneuver, the dog remained difficult to ventilate.

A catheter was inserted into the dorsal pedal artery for continuously monitoring arterial blood pressure and periodic sampling of arterial blood for blood gas analysis. Because of her low plasma protein, dextran 70 was started in addition to lactated Ringer's solution. After surgical preparation the dog was moved to the OR.

Once positioned in dorsal recumbency and while breathing spontaneously, an arterial blood sample was collected for blood gas analysis; the results were: pH 7.22, $P_a CO_2$ 55 mmHg, $P_a O_2$ 51 mmHg, standard base excess −5.1 mEq L^{-1}. Mean arterial blood pressure was 105 mmHg, heart rate was 120 beats per minute, SpO$_2$ was 89%, and $P_E'CO_2$ was 39 mmHg.

The surgeon made a ventral abdominal midline incision. As soon as the abdominal cavity was entered, all evidence of the dog's ventilation ceased in that the reservoir bag stopped moving and the capnograph went to zero. Mechanical ventilation was initiated and the anesthetist asked the surgeon to check the dog's diaphragm. The diaphragm had a rent in it with portions of the liver including the gallbladder and omentum extending through the rent into the thoracic cavity. The thoracic cavity was tapped and 100 mL of serous fluid was removed. After a median sternotomy was performed to gain better access to the thoracic cavity, an additional 2 L of fluid was removed and further exploration revealed a torsion of the right middle lung lobe. Fibrinous, purulent material floating freely in the abdomen was assumed to be the "puppy." Because of the dog's unstable condition under anesthesia the surgeon decided to close the chest, leaving resolution of the lung lobe torsion to a later date (performed 8 days later). Anesthesia lasted 125 minutes. The dog was recovered in an oxygen cage in the ICU where the remainder of her recovery and analgesia were managed.

Initial analysis of the case

The dog obviously had a diaphragmatic hernia, but some elements of the case at presentation led the receiving veterinarian to make an initial diagnosis of dystocia. The owner's history of the dog and her opinion that the dog was trying to deliver puppies, certainly set the stage for this diagnosis. There was also confirmation of this diagnosis by the radiologist, and the limited blood work provided additional, seemingly confirmatory evidence. The hematocrit was 31% and total plasma solids were 5.8 g dL^{-1}, numbers that are expected in a bitch at term. However, the blood glucose of 3.83 mmol L^{-1} was low and, at the very least, suggested that the dog had an inadequate diet.

For the anesthetist managing this patient, details of the history and physical examination, including the nervous and aggressive nature of the bitch and her unkempt hair coat, the latter finding suggesting she was not well cared for, all suggested that something was amiss. This was not a typical at-term patient. The anesthetist's experience in managing anesthesia for numerous caesarean deliveries was that most bitches with dystocia are not aggressive, even during abdominal palpation. In fact, most of them presenting for emergency caesarean delivery are quite manageable, possibly because of exhaustion, dehydration, and lack of sleep.

Had there been better communication between anesthesia and surgery, had they functioned as one team instead of two seemingly antagonistic teams, the patient and the client would have been much better served. Indeed, had there been better communication between the services (including radiology), and a sharing of information, observations, and findings about the bitch's condition, a more thorough understanding of her condition may have developed.

A complete blood count (CBC) probably would have indicated that this dog had an ongoing inflammatory process. However, knowing that there would be a delay in obtaining the CBC results along with concerns about the well-being of the puppy and a sense of urgency to get the dog to surgery, probably would have led both teams to relegate this blood work to the bottom of the to-do list. However, a radiograph of the abdomen, especially if it included the caudal portion of the thorax, would have been very informative. Radiographs would have ruled in or ruled out the presence of a fetus by revealing its skeletal structure, which at term would be obvious. Ultrasound, especially in an uncooperative and aggressive animal, is not necessarily diagnostic in a case such as this.

None of these steps were considered and the true diagnosis only became apparent at the beginning of surgery.

Investigation of the case

A diagnostic error occurred early in this case, but it was then exacerbated by breakdowns in communications. The dog's history of having been hit by a car 5 months previously was important, but the owner was not questioned further concerning that event. No one in the veterinary team dealing with the case knew if the dog had been taken to a local veterinarian for workup and treatment after being hit by the car, or had recovered on her own at home. This historical entry about the accident was treated as an historical aside and given

little importance in the overall assessment of the dog. However, opportunities to correct this initial mistake were missed due to other errors.

The environment in which we work (the context) affects patient care either positively or negatively. In this case there was an ongoing tension between the surgery and anesthesia services due to a perception by the surgery service that anesthesia intentionally delayed its cases. These tensions led to poor interdisciplinary communication and teamwork and as a consequence patient care was suboptimal and the client was not well served.

This case has some features in common with the polar bear case (see Case 6.1 in Chapter 6). In both cases the veterinarians became fixated on what seemed to be each patient's primary problem, whether it was fractures or dystocia, and did so without considering other problems that were in fact present and to which a number of signs strongly pointed. In other words, a fixation bias existed.

Both cases also present what could be called the "visiting professional trap." In the case of the polar bear, the zoo veterinarian was an outsider to the referral hospital's anesthesia and surgical team. Out of professional courtesy and in recognition of his expertise with the medical care of zoo animals, that team did not question what turned out to be an incomplete diagnosis despite many signs pointing to serious internal injuries. In this case of the pregnant bitch, the visiting professional trap was the visiting veterinary radiologist.

During rounds at which this case was discussed, it was discovered that the visiting radiologist was inexperienced in ultrasonography and was visiting the practice to gain additional training in this imaging technique. On the day this patient presented for ultrasound examination the supervising ultrasonographer in charge of training the visiting radiologist, was off the clinic floor and unavailable to review the case. So what's the lesson? Amongst colleagues—whether known or strangers—it is always acceptable to question a diagnosis and how it was arrived at. Yes, such questioning should be done in a collegial manner, but when the circumstances so indicate, thoughtful, probing questioning is appropriate.

The dog had a diaphragmatic hernia, a diagnosis that ties together so many clues in the history and physical examination. It is also apparent that the uncollegial environment of this practice at that time precluded a team approach to patient management. A functional team probably would have been better able to sort through this patient's history and physical examination so as to make a medical diagnosis as opposed to an unexpected surgical finding.

Case 7.2

A 10-year-old, 6-kg, spayed domestic longhair cat was taken to a specialty ophthalmology practice by its owner, whose chief complaint was that the cat's pupils were dilated and unresponsive to light. During physical examination the cat was found to have bilateral bullous retinal detachment and intraretinal non-tapetal hemorrhage in the left eye. Further physical examination did not detect other abnormalities except for a mild bradycardia (150 beats per minute). Systolic blood pressures were measured indirectly with a Doppler blood pressure device and were within normal limits (~123 mmHg). After starting treatment for the eye condition with prednisone and methazolamide, the cat was sent home. The owner brought the cat back the next day for laser repair of the bilateral retinal detachment.

A complete blood count showed clinically insignificant changes in the hemogram and the only abnormality in an endocrine panel was a low total T4 but T3 within normal limits. Chest radiographs indicated that the lungs had a mild, diffuse increase in opacity along airways, which created parallel lines and rings. No other abnormalities were detected and the radiology resident, who read the radiographs, stated that the cause and clinical significance of the mild diffuse airway lung pattern was uncertain, but could be due to inflammatory or immune-mediated airway disease, cardiogenic or non-cardiogenic pulmonary edema, or possibly infiltrative neoplasia; cardiomegaly was not observed.

On the day of surgery the cat was blind but behaviorally alert, active, and responsive. She was premedicated with a combination of hydromorphone and midazolam, both injected intramuscularly. Approximately 10 minutes later she was sufficiently sedated for intravenous catheterization. After pre-oxygenating the cat for 5 minutes, she was induced to anesthesia with a mixture of thiopental and propofol. Immediately after induction the cat was intubated and anesthesia was maintained with isoflurane in oxygen. The eyes were lubricated with bland petrolatum ointment, and standard monitoring was instituted, including electrocardiogram, expired CO_2, and a Doppler for indirect systolic arterial blood pressure. A pulse oximeter probe was placed on the tongue, and isotonic fluids were administered intravenously. The electrocardiogram showed a sinus rhythm of 110 beats per minute, and oxygen saturation was 100%. The first blood pressure reading indicated a systolic pressure of 80 mmHg; the isoflurane vaporizer dial setting was reduced. A second catheter was inserted into the right cephalic vein for administering additional fluids should they be needed. Systolic blood pressure increased to 100 mmHg and the patient seemed stable and sufficiently anesthetized to be transported to the ophthalmology treatment area for laser repair of the bilateral retinal detachment.

Surgery proceeded uneventfully. During the procedure systolic blood pressure ranged between 100 and 110 mmHg, and heart rate was around 100 beats per minute. The patient breathed spontaneously for the duration of anesthesia with a respiratory rate of 8 breaths per minute; expired CO_2 ranged between 44 and 46 mmHg. After the procedure was completed the cat was returned to the induction area where the isoflurane was discontinued, and the cat was awakened.

Fifteen minutes later the cat was extubated; her rectal temperature was 35 °C, so the anesthesia team decided to keep the patient between two circulating warm water heating pads and under a Bair Hugger™ blanket until her temperature reached 36.1 °C. No analgesics were administered postoperatively because the patient seemed comfortable. While the cat was being warmed, the ophthalmology student extern assigned to the patient was asked to go to the ophthalmology surgical suite to assist with another case. Normally the ophthalmology extern would stay with the patient assigned to his or her care and would do so in the ophthalmology ward until the patient was normothermic and fully recovered from anesthesia. Since the cat was not normothermic a decision was made to keep it in the anesthesia recovery area rather than return it to the ward. Within a few minutes the cat's temperature was 36.1 °C and it was moved to one of the anesthesia recovery room cages; the Bair Hugger™ was used to continue warming the cat by blowing warm air into the cage.

Because the anesthesia schedule was full and busy, the anesthetist assigned to the cat was told to start another case. It was agreed, however, that someone would check the cat's temperature in a few minutes. Approximately 3 hours later the cat was found unresponsive in the recovery room cage; the Bair Hugger™ was still in operation. Cardiopulmonary resuscitation

(CPR) was initiated, but after 10 minutes of effort it was discontinued since cardiac electrical activity and peripheral pulses could not be detected, and the pupils were dilated and fixed.

The cat was necropsied later that day. The gross pathologic findings were mild hypertrophic cardiomyopathy and patchy pulmonary hemorrhage and edema. Histopathology indicated that the right and left ventricles and the interventricular septum were within normal limits; the pulmonary changes were described as acute pulmonary hemorrhage and edema. The eyes had lymphoplasmacytic anterior uveitis and ciliary lymphocytic neuritis.

Initial analysis of the case

An anesthesia schedule coordinates the many elements that bring together the patient, the clinician performing the procedure whatever it may be, the anesthetist, the facilities and the equipment to perform all necessary procedures. In a large multi-veterinarian practice many diverse services often simultaneously request anesthesia support, a reality that causes production pressures involving demands on time, resources, and energy, and creates distractions. It is well recognized in the nuclear and aviation industries that errors are more likely to occur in busy, stressful environments (Wheeler & Wheeler 2005). In this particular case both the anesthesia and ophthalmology services were busy and short-staffed. As a result the anesthetist and the student ophthalmology extern assigned to this particular patient had to attend to other patients thus leaving this patient unattended.

The cat died in the post-anesthesia period at a time when the anesthetist was concerned about the cat's hypothermia, a condition known to be a source of complications in this particular practice as well as the wider veterinary community (Brodbelt *et al.* 2007, 2008). The death was unwitnessed and occurred at a time when the cat should have been under observation. Clarke and Hall (1990) showed that many of the anesthesia-related deaths reported in their study occurred at a time when the dogs and cats were not under close observation. In this case, it is clear that an important role, that of monitoring the patient in recovery, was not assigned to a specific person. Although the patient's death may not have been prevented, it is likely that had someone been assigned to monitor the patient in recovery, he or she would have noticed a deterioration in its condition and initiated an investigation and intervened as necessary.

Investigation of the case

Two factors played a primary role in this incident: (1) a failure to manage personnel resources in that no one was specifically designated to routinely and periodically check the cat; (2) even if someone had been clearly identified to check the cat throughout the recovery phase there was no mechanism in place to remind that person or anyone else in the induction area, to periodically check the cat.

The first error is a failure in communication and teamwork. For a team to work effectively roles have to be clearly defined and communicated. In this case not only was the task of monitoring the cat in recovery not prioritized, it was overlooked—omitted—and the task was not assigned to anyone. Normally it would be the extern's job to monitor the patient in recovery, but it should be kept in mind that, however competent externs may be, they are in fact visiting students or staff who probably are not fully cognizant of the system and their role within it. On this note, care should always be taken whenever externs, students, or new staff members are given clinical responsibility as errors are likely to occur if roles are not well defined and communicated clearly and regularly. When asked to go to another surgery by the service the extern was visiting, it is not surprising that the cat was left solely with anesthesia, which was also stretched to its limits by the busy schedule. The anesthetist in charge of the case should have passed on the information and instructions concerning this cat to another staff member, but it is easy to see that under demands of a busy schedule these details were overlooked.

This brings us to the second error: lack of a memory-jogging cue. This error gets to the heart of the reality of short-term memory; it is the most labile of human memory (Reason 1990). Any factor that distracts someone from the task at hand has the potential to cause an error known as a capture slip. In this case, without an effective memory-jogging mechanism in place, the busy schedule almost assured that no member of the team involved with this patient would remember to check on it.

What specific elements should have been in place to make certain the cat was periodically checked? The procedure put in effect after this adverse incident provides a possible solution, one that addresses two of the issues that have been discussed so far. The process that was put in place involved creating and dedicating a column on the anesthesia scheduling board for patients recovering from anesthesia. When a patient is recovering from anesthesia, its schedule ticket and a recovery form are moved to the recovery column at the head of which is the name of the person who is responsible for checking recovering patients. The recovery form is used to monitor and record the time when vital signs, such as heart and respiratory rates and rectal temperature, are checked so as to assess a patient's recovery. A patient can be moved to a ward cage only after several parameters are met: rectal temperature is 37.2–39.2 °C; the patient is awake and aware (tracks movement and sound), moves on its own, and has minimal if any pain. When these parameters are met, the patient is deemed successfully recovered from anesthesia, and the time and ward to which the patient is moved are recorded on the form, which becomes part of the patient's medical record.

Although the exact reason for the cat's demise remains a mystery (perhaps fluid overload or heat stress?) it is clear that with better teamwork and communication the cat would not have been left unobserved for 3 hours.

Case 7.3

A 10-year-old, 20-kg male beagle was presented for castration. With little advanced warning, the internal medicine resident who admitted the dog had asked that it be squeezed into the anesthesia-surgery schedule as a "day case" because it belonged to an extremely good client who had been bringing the dog to the hospital's oncology service for many years. The dog had been undergoing treatment for low-grade lymphoma, for which it was in remission. It also had mild mitral valve disease and had recently developed prostatic hyperplasia, hence the need for castration. According to the notes for the dog's current visit it was not on medications, a fact confirmed on the anesthetic request form. Unfortunately the dog's complete paper file was missing and the hospital's computer records, designed primarily for purposes of billing, contained only brief notes about diagnosis, interventions, and treatments performed at the hospital, so they provided little additional information.

At examination the dog was bright and alert, and apart from the grade II/VI soft systolic heart murmur over the mitral valve, no significant abnormalities were detected; heart rate was 96 beats per minute with a sinus arrhythmia. Pulse quality was good.

An anesthetic plan was prepared and approved, and a catheter was inserted into a cephalic vein (the dog was well trained for this procedure). Acepromazine and methadone were subsequently slowly administered intravenously. After 2 minutes the dog collapsed. Clinical examination revealed signs of cardiovascular collapse. Heart rate was 55 beats per minute, peripheral pulses were poor, mucous membranes were pale with a prolonged capillary refill time. An electrocardiogram showed a sinus bradycardia and an oscillometric blood pressure reading revealed blood pressures of 88/40 [63] mmHg (systolic/diastolic [mean arterial] blood pressure). As no other cause was apparent it was assumed the dog had a vasovagal collapse.

Atropine was administered intravenously, which increased the heart rate and blood pressure to more acceptable levels; the dog improved over the next 30 minutes. Anesthesia was continued after an hour of delay so as to allow the dog to recover and to ensure further mishaps would not occur. Anesthesia was induced with alfaxalone and maintained with sevoflurane in oxygen. Each testicle was injected with lidocaine and the sevoflurane vaporizer setting was maintained at 1% throughout anesthesia. Ephedrine was administered intravenously once to maintain mean arterial blood pressure above 70 mmHg and to increase heart rate, which had decreased slightly during the surgical preparation phase. The surgery went well and the patient recovered uneventfully.

When transferring the patient from the recovery room to the internal medicine ward the receiving technician asked: "When is the next dose of benazepril due?" No mention had ever been made to the anesthetist that the dog was receiving benazepril. Had this fact been known, another premedicant other than acepromazine, would have been selected. Furthermore, after receiving the acepromazine, at least 8 hours would have had to elapse before additional benazepril could be administered.

Investigation

It was confirmed that the dog was indeed on medications, specifically the angiotensin converting enzyme inhibitor benazepril for management of its mitral valve disease. The internal medicine resident who had admitted the dog, had asked the owners about any medications the dog was receiving, but failed to write that information down on either the paper history form or anesthetic request form. The information had been put on the dog's cage sheet, but these sheets stayed in the ward on the animal's cage and were not taken to the anesthetic induction room. In fact, the medicine resident thought this medication detail was irrelevant to the surgical procedure the dog was to undergo, so did not pass it on. When asked about the omission, the resident said that they were busy and should not have been asked to admit an oncology patient for surgery.

Eventually the dog's clinical file was found in the oncologist's office, where it had been since the dog's visit the previous week. The file clearly outlined the dog's current medication history. The benazepril had been started by the referring veterinarian as the owners had wanted to "do something" about the dog's heart murmur. For this reason the drug did not appear on the hospital's computerized record system.

Analysis

This is a classic case of communication source failure (see "Communication: what it is and how it fails" in Chapter 2) in that information was not passed on to the people who needed to know it. This type of error probably occurs daily in most practices. In this case both oral and written communications were faulty. In the hospital of this case there are sections in both the paper history form and paper anesthetic request form for current medications, but neither were completed in this case. Furthermore, the anesthetic request form is supposed to be accompanied by a verbal request made to the anesthetist in charge of the day's list of cases. In this case the verbal request was brief as it was made by the technician who brought the dog to anesthesia; the medicine resident who admitted the patient was busy attending to another patient. The case moved ahead as the surgeon had been informed by the oncologist that the dog may arrive for surgery without having been admitted through the usual admission process (something the owners tended to do!), and had already discussed the case with the anesthetist. Of course, not having admitted the patient, the surgeon, too, did not possess all the facts pertaining to it.

The missing medical records compounded this problem as there was no way the anesthetist could have known that the dog was receiving any medications. Paper medical records can be cumbersome and are prone to information loss (often due to parts or all of the record being lost). Paper medical records may be considered somewhat old-fashioned today, but even if a hospital uses electronic medical records, it is not unusual for some information, such as anesthetic records, day sheets, and charts, to be paper-based. When two such systems exist, it means there is the potential for failure to transfer information from the paper form to the computerized record and for it to be potentially lost. Whenever information about a patient is lost, whatever the cause, there is the chance that an error will occur. Electronic medical records should improve communication between clinicians about patients, but their success depends on accurate and complete transfer of patient information into the system.

There was also a significant lack of teamwork in this case, insofar as the resident admitting the patient did less than a thorough job. The resident felt that the responsibility for the case did not "belong to them" and did not believe it was "their job" to admit the patient. If the resident was indeed busy, this sentiment is understandable, but the resident should have made this clear and asked for another clinician to admit the case rather than admit the case in a sub-standard fashion. To be fair, the resident knew very little about the patient and begrudgingly admitted the dog only because the surgeon was in the operating room and unavailable, and the senior oncologist in charge of the patient was away. The resident also had little experience in admitting patients for surgery. Nonetheless, the lack of teamwork was disappointing and perhaps reflected a lack of interdisciplinary courtesy and cooperation, a situation that may be all too common in multidisciplinary hospitals.

Near miss vignette

Vignette 7.1

During a busy day of orthopedic cases an anesthetist, before setting up for the next patient, calls the wards area and requests that the next patient be premedicated. When asked which patient, the anesthetist informs the technician that it is a "dog due to get a TTT."

Half an hour later a request is made to bring the dog to the anesthesia room. The anesthetist helps a student insert an intravenous catheter into the dog's cephalic vein and then requests that a technician assist the student with induction. Prior to induction the technician performs a pre-anesthetic checklist. When the dog's name is checked against the anesthesia-surgery schedule its name differs from that of the patient that is suppose to be anesthetized at that time for surgery. The dog was due to undergo a TTT procedure (tibial tuberosity transposition for patellar luxation) whereas the dog actually scheduled to be next on the anesthesia-surgery schedule was to undergo a TTA (tibial tuberosity advancement for cranial cruciate rupture) procedure. The anesthetist admitted not knowing the difference between the two procedures. Although the scheduling kerfuffle needed some smoothing over with the owners of the two dogs (and with the orthopedic surgeon!), it did not cause harm to the patients, just a reshuffling of the order of cases.

In this situation two communication problems are identifiable. Firstly, the failure to use the animal's name to clearly identify it. It is too easy to communicate a patient's identity using its signalment and illness or procedure. Although often easier to remember than a name, using such generic descriptors is more likely to lead to cases of mistaken identity. Even designations like "Ben the Labrador" can be problematic as it is quite likely that two dogs with the same name could be hospitalized at the same time. Although it may appear to be longwinded, using an animal's name, client's last name, and a unique identification number is the ideal way of identifying patients.

Secondly, the use of abbreviations. Abbreviations have become the unofficial shorthand of medical and veterinary communications because they simplify and accelerate communications. Unfortunately, each specialty has evolved its own collection of abbreviations for common, specialty-specific terms, often done so in isolation, and these shorthand techniques may not be recognizable to those working in different disciplines (Parvaiz et al. 2008). Parvaiz studied how well a multidisciplinary group of clinicians could identify abbreviations found in orthopedic medical records in a single hospital (Parvaiz et al. 2008). Even orthopedic surgeons could only correctly identify 57% of the abbreviations! From this it is clear that abbreviations hinder communications; the use of unfamiliar abbreviations causes misunderstandings and frustration, and detracts from the meaning of the information being transmitted. Abbreviations may also have multiple meanings depending on context, and the context may only be known to the person transmitting the information. For example, "AUS" may mean "abdominal ultrasound scan" or "artificial urethral sphincter." This could be

problematic as an animal undergoing an artificial urethral sphincter procedure may also have an abdominal ultrasound examination performed. When the anesthesia service is approached about a schedule slot for a bitch with urinary incontinence the abbreviation will not, without further elaboration, describe the procedure the bitch is to undergo. Most studies investigating the use of abbreviations, in various medical fields, suggest that abbreviations should be used sparingly and only for terms recognized between the transmitter and receiver of information. In fact, the Joint Commission on the Accreditation of Healthcare Organizations has developed a "Do Not Use" list of abbreviations due to findings that 5% of medication errors reported to the US Pharmacopeia MEDMARX national medication error reporting program, were caused by the use of abbreviations (Brunetti 2007). All of this suggests, at the very least, that veterinary hospitals or practices should create an agreed list of abbreviations for internal communications. Better yet would be the elimination of abbreviations in our communications.

Conclusion

The ability to communicate and manage resources effectively involves what are referred to as non-technical skills. Without a doubt these are important skills in medical practice (Fletcher et al. 2003; Larsson & Holmström 2013; Rutherford et al. 2012), but the term "non-technical skills" has a bit of a "touchy-feely" connotation to it, one that seems to imply that these skills are "poor cousins" to technical skills.

These cases, however, present some of the ways in which breakdowns in communications and resource management—non-technical skills—can adversely affect patient care, or disrupt the flow of patient management in veterinary medicine.

Every method of communication is prone to error. Oral communications are often only partially recalled by the receiver. Written communications are time consuming so are often only partially completed. Electronic communications are often too brief. No single method of communicating information between individuals and teams in veterinary medicine is infallible, which suggests that information be transmitted in multiple ways. Forms should be backed up with verbal communications and vice versa. To be well understood, communication should be simple and direct (but friendly and collegial), be free from ambiguity and jargon, and be as concise as possible. Standardizing communication and communication training should be encouraged.

References

Brindley, P.G. (2014) I. Improving teamwork in anaesthesia and critical care: Many lessons still to learn. *British Journal of Anaesthesia* **112**(3): 399–401.

Brodbelt, D.C., *et al.* (2007) Risk factors for anaesthetic-related death in cats: Results from the Confidential Enquiry into Perioperative Small Animal Fatalities (CEPSAF). *British Journal of Anaesthesia* **99**(5): 617–623.

Brodbelt, D.C., *et al.* (2008) Results of the Confidential Enquiry into Perioperative Small Animal Fatalities regarding risk factors for anaesthetic-related death in dogs. *Journal of the American Veterinary Medical Association* **233**(7): 1096–1104.

Brunetti, L. (2007) Abbreviations formally linked to medication errors. *Healthcare Benchmarks and Quality Improvement* **14**(11): 126–128.

Bunting, R.F. Jr & Groszkruger, D.P. (2016) From to err is human to improving diagnosis in health care: The risk management perspective. *Journal of Healthcare Risk Management* **35**(3): 10–23.

Clarke, K.W. & Hall, L.W. (1990) A survey of anaesthesia in small animal practice: AVA/BSAVA report. *Veterinary Anaesthesia and Analgesia* **17**: 4–10.

Fletcher, G., *et al.* (2003) Anaesthetists' Non-Technical skills (ANTS): Evaluation of a behavioural marker system. *British Journal of Anaesthesia* **90**(5): 580–588.

Greenberg, C.C., *et al.* (2007) Patterns of communication breakdowns resulting in injury to surgical patients. *Journal of the American College of Surgeons* **204**(4): 533–540.

Kinnison, T., *et al.* (2015) Errors in veterinary practice: Preliminary lessons for building better veterinary teams. *Veterinary Record* **177**(19): 492.

Larsson, J. & Holmström, I.K. (2013) How excellent anaesthetists perform in the operating theatre: A qualitative study on non-technical skills. *British Journal of Anaesthesia* **110**(1): 115–121.

Lingard, L., *et al.* (2004) Communication failures in the operating room: An observational classification of recurrent types and effects. *Quality & Safety in Health Care* **13**(5): 330–334.

Nagpal, K., *et al.* (2012) Failures in communication and information transfer across the surgical care pathway: Interview study. *BMJ Quality & Safety* **21**(10): 843–849.

Oxtoby, C., *et al.* (2015) We need to talk about error: Causes and types of error in veterinary practice. *Veterinary Record* **177**(17): 438–445.

Parvaiz, M.A., *et al.* (2008) The use of abbreviations in medical records in a multidisciplinary world—an imminent disaster. *Communication & Medicine* **5**(1): 25–33.

Reason, J.T. (1990) *Human Error*. Cambridge: Cambridge University Press.

Rutherford, J.S., *et al.* (2012) Non-technical skills of anaesthetic assistants in the perioperative period: A literature review. *British Journal of Anaesthesia* **109**(1): 27–31.

Salas, E., *et al.* (2008) Communicating, coordinating, and cooperating when lives depend on it: Tips for teamwork. *Joint Commission Journal on Quality and Patient Safety/Joint Commission Resources* **34**(6): 333–341.

Weick, K.E. (2002) The reduction of medical errors through mindful interdependence. In: *Medical Errors: What Do We Know? What Do We Do?* (eds M.M. Rosenthal & K.M. Sutcliffe), 1st edn. San Francisco, CA: Jossey-Bass, pp. 177–199.

Wheeler, S.J. & Wheeler, D.W. (2005) Medication errors in anaesthesia and critical care. *Anaesthesia* **60**(3): 257–273.

CHAPTER 8

Error Prevention in Veterinary Anesthesia

To give safety a future, we should not see people as a problem to control, but as a solution we can harness. We need to move from counting negatives to understanding what makes an organization normally successful. And we need the courage to question common wisdom and industry standards—confronting fiction with facts, and faith with enlightenment.

Sydney Dekker, Safety Differently: Human Factors for a New Era, 2013

Tell me and I forget, teach me and I may remember, involve me and I learn.

Benjamin Franklin

Insanity is doing the same thing over and over again and expecting different results.

Albert Einstein

There are two ways in which safety can be viewed as a process, a goal to be achieved. The classical view approaches it reactively in that when an error occurs actions are taken to prevent further errors by stopping bad stuff from happening, that is, by eliminating the negative. This approach can be very effective, as demonstrated by the aviation industry with its standards and guidelines and record of safety. This approach addresses safety incidents by introducing control measures, such as guidelines and standard operating procedures (SOPs), in the hope of altering the system so as to reduce the chances of similar errors occurring in the future. Indeed, when implemented appropriately, standardization plays a key role in developing safe practices because collective expertise and experiences are recorded and formally passed on to those involved with the process. But poorly thought out and implemented standard operating procedures can give the impression of furthering safety in one area while actually increasing the risk of unsafe acts occurring in another. Box 8.1 gives an example from a university veterinary teaching hospital that serves to make this point.

As the example in Box 8.1 suggests, the reactive approach, at least in medicine, is probably not always the best approach, in part because of the uncertainty and ambiguity prevalent throughout clinical medicine, surgery, and anesthesia. Situations arise in which the patient does not fit the circumstances that a control

> **Box 8.1** Example of an unforeseen risk associated with implementation of a "safe" policy for handling of hypodermic needles.
>
> A hospital encounters many needle-stick injuries due to staff and students resheathing hypodermic needles prior to their safe disposal. Hospital management takes the seemingly logical step of banning all resheathing of needles; staff and students are trained in methods of removing needles without resheathing. This new policy is emphasized and reinforced regularly through emails and poster campaigns. The number of needle-stick injuries due to resheathing decreases substantially. Unfortunately, as a result of this policy people with unsheathed needles are observed wandering around the clinic trying to find a sharps container for safe disposal of the needles. The top-down approach to the problem did not consider the importance of having sharps containers available at locations where needles are likely to be used. As a result a second more problematic risk has been introduced: instead of people sticking themselves, they risked sticking others. The original risk has been managed, but the risk of needle sticks has merely shifted to a different set of people.

measure or standard operating procedure was designed to address. Guidelines or standardized processes cannot account for all conditions and circumstances that a veterinarian may encounter when anesthetizing a patient because, at the very least, anesthesia always perturbs a

Errors in Veterinary Anesthesia, First Edition. John W. Ludders and Matthew McMillan.

patient's normal physiology and every patient and each anesthetic is different.

An alternate view of safety as a goal is one that is proactive and strives to maximize the chances of success, accentuating the positive to ensure that "good stuff happens." Safety in this light is the ability to succeed under varying conditions, regardless of ambiguity or uncertainty, so that the number of intended and acceptable outcomes is as high as possible (Hollnagel 2014). Success in anesthesia is not merely having an awake and alive patient at the end of the anesthetic, but means that all processes in the anesthesia procedure were managed with attention to patient safety. Given this definition of success, unsafe practices, even when the outcomes are "successful," are still unsafe and unacceptable; success following unsafe practices may be due to nothing more than modern anesthetic drugs and equipment, or worse yet, mere chance. The number and severity of near misses that may have occurred as a result of unsafe practices may, on another day and under different circumstances, become harmful hits. Success in safety terms means that an outcome was achieved by actively striving for patient safety throughout the procedure. How do we achieve this?

A first step is to acknowledge that errors do occur in anesthesia and then focus on patient safety as a goal of the organization, of individuals within the organization, and with regards to technical factors. We also need to recognize that most of us tend to be overconfident in our cognitive abilities while often denigrating the use of cognitive aids, such as checklists, calculators, standard operating procedures, and guidelines; often we hear that such aids are only "for poor clinicians." Once these realities are recognized and accepted it becomes easier to take actions that focus on achieving patient safety in the daily practice of medicine, surgery, or anesthesia. The next sections present some general and some specific strategies for achieving this goal. The general strategies include suggestions for bringing about changes in behaviors and habits that foster patient safety, and the attributes of effective anesthetists. More specific strategies include: identifying elements that should be part of a "safety culture"; minimizing distractions; cognitive forcing strategies; breaking our reliance on memory by using cognitive aids such as checklists and mnemonics; strategies for improving communication and teamwork; and methods for evaluating the processes of anesthesia and redesigning them with safety in mind.

General strategies for error prevention

Changing habits: getting away from "We've always done it that way"

Although the idea of improving safety (minimizing error) by changing our practices would appear to be a no-brainer, it is easier said than done. Enforcing change through a top-down approach rarely works; it puts our collective backs up and breeds resentment. In the face of change too often we hear: "What's wrong with how we're doing things now?" "What's the point of this? It's a waste of time," "We didn't have a problem before, what's the issue now?", "If it ain't broke, don't fix it," or even "Who are they to tell me how to do my job!" All are common retorts whenever anything new gets introduced to a well-entrenched system. Experience and studies have shown that changes are more likely to be integrated into practice if the people performing the tasks are involved in the decision-making and implementation processes (Roberts *et al.* 2005; Vogus & Hilligoss 2015). Most people want and need to know why something has to be changed before they will accept that it should be changed. So the process starts by informing staff as to why change is necessary, by describing the problems that are being encountered. Openness and reporting of real data—facts on the ground—are key components of this process.

Once frontline staff recognize there are problems within the system in which they work the next step is to involve them in the change process. This can be achieved by encouraging staff to take ownership of the work by allowing them to be responsible for making improvements in their areas of expertise. There are processes by which this can be accomplished, one of which is outlined in the Theoretical Domains Framework (Michie *et al.* 2005) that can be used to assess a target group's knowledge, skills, beliefs about their capabilities, motivation, goals, and behavior; it presents questions the group should ask itself when considering implementing a change in some X process, which could be a procedure or a protocol (Table 8.1). Of crucial importance is that this framework is not used solely by management as it considers making a change, but is used by the target group itself as it assesses its attributes and abilities to make a change. It is not a top-down process, it is an inclusive process. The answers to the questions in the framework help guide the group as to how to effect the necessary changes.

Table 8.1 The following can serve as a guide for implementing an evidence-based practice. The domains and questions that should be asked and answered help to make sure that processes both favoring and opposing implementation are identified so that the change in practice can be implemented successfully.

Domains	Questions to ask
Knowledge	Do they know about the guideline?
	What do they think the evidence is?
Skills	Do they know how to do X?
	How easy or difficult do they find performing X?
Social/professional role and identity	What is the purpose of X?
	Do they think guidelines should determine their behavior?
	Is doing X compatible or in conflict with professional standards/identity? (prompts: moral/ethical issues, limits to autonomy)
Beliefs about capabilities	How capable are they of maintaining X?
Beliefs about consequences (anticipated outcomes/attitude)	What do they think will happen if they do X? (prompt re themselves, patients, colleagues, and organization; positive and negative, short- and long-term consequences)
	What are the costs of X and what are the costs of the consequences of X?
Motivation and goals	How much do they want to do X?
	Are there other things they want to do or achieve that might interfere with X?
	Does the guideline conflict with others?
	Are there incentives to do X?
Memory, attention, and decision processes	Is X something they usually do?
	Will they think to do X?
	How much attention will they have to pay to do X?
	Will they remember to do X?
Environmental context and resources (environmental constraints)	To what extent do physical or resource factors facilitate or hinder X?
	Are there competing tasks and time constraints?
	Are the necessary resources available to those expected to undertake X?
Social influences (norms)	To what extent do social influences facilitate or hinder X? (prompts: peers, managers, other professional groups, patients, relatives)
Emotion	Does doing X evoke an emotional response? If so, what?
	To what extent do emotional factors facilitate or hinder X?
Behavioral regulation	What preparatory steps are needed to do X? (prompt re individual and organizational)
	Are there procedures or ways of working that encourage X?
Nature of the behavior	What is the proposed behavior (X)?
	Who needs to do what differently when, where, how, how often, and with whom?
	Is this a new behavior or an existing behavior that needs to become a habit?
	Can the context be used to prompt the new behavior? (prompts: layout, reminders, equipment)
	How long are changes going to take?
	Are there systems for maintaining long-term change?

Adapted from: Michie, S., Johnston, M., Abraham, C., *et al.* (2005) Making psychological theory useful for implementing evidence based practice: a consensus approach. *Quality & Safety in Health Care* **14**(1): 26–33. With permission of the publisher.

Attributes of an effective anesthetist

An effective anesthetist is one who understands that "to err is human" and realizes that errors and accidents will occur in anesthesia; one who recognizes that anesthetists work in complex settings and situations. But what are the characteristics of an effective anesthetist, one who functions effectively in such circumstances? To answer this question we draw on the work of Klemola and Norros, and Reason. The former two have identified essential characteristics of effective anesthetists. They believe that an anesthetist's perception of a given situation within a clinical context is inseparable from the anesthetist's history and behavioral profile (Klemola 2000; Norros & Klemola 1999). They contend that because anesthesia is filled with inherent uncertainty it is necessary to consider the situated character of human activity and that anesthetists' habits of action should be explored within those particular circumstances in which they use their resources, that is, within the operating room. Because anesthesia has inherent uncertainty, Klemola and Norros do not believe it is an activity that can be governed by general rules or rigid guidelines. Indeed, they believe that to do so ignores the dynamic nature of anesthesia and a patient's responses during anesthesia (Klemola 2000; Klemola & Norros 1997, 2001; Norros & Klemola 1999).

Klemola and Norros believe that to cope with the uncertainties of anesthesia, the anesthetist must use judgment based on efficient interpretation and use of situational information (Klemola & Norros 1997; Norros & Klemola 1999). Klemola further argues that the use of training techniques such as those used in the aviation industry, may be inappropriate in anesthesia because they are based on the assumption that anesthetists and pilots use similar "mental models," an assumption Klemola believes is unfounded (Klemola 2000). Furthermore, the belief that general rules can be used to guide the anesthetist in the practice of anesthesia is possible only when the human mind is viewed as an information processing mechanism (a computer) that follows computational rules (Cook & Woods 1994), a view with which Klemola disagrees (Klemola 2000). The problem of likening the brain to a computer ignores the complexity of the brain and the reality that our brains, unlike computers, are affected by many factors, such as emotions, fatigue, distractions of all sorts, and factors that can degrade our short-term memory and affect our perceptions of and interactions with the real world. Furthermore, unlike transforming computer code into an application, it is difficult to transform knowledge into practice because neither general rules nor specific clinical recommendations include instructions on how to apply them in the everyday fuzzy and unruly situations so often encountered in anesthesia. The nature of knowledge is also a problem in that a valid statistical fact does not say much about a particular patient, especially when there is so much inherent uncertainty that cannot be governed by general rules (Norros & Klemola 1999). A single statistic certainly does not describe the total context within which an anesthetist works.

The effective anesthetist must detect and respond to an incident, and it is the dynamic complexity of anesthesia that sets specific requirements for the anesthetist's activities including the manner in which he or she views the patient (Klemola & Norros 1997). In their studies of the clinical behavior of expert anesthetists, Klemola and Norros identified two distinct behavioral profiles (Klemola & Norros 1997; Norros & Klemola 1999):

1 The **interpretive profile** in which the anesthetist clearly and efficiently uses situationally relevant information based on insights of the patient's physiological responses to anesthesia, especially during the induction phase of anesthesia. The anesthetist's actions are guided by an understanding of the uniqueness and uncertainty of actual situations, and effectively and skillfully uses anesthetic drugs or monitor-derived information.

2 The **objectivistic profile** in which the anesthetist views the patient as a natural object and uncertainty is not recognized; the anesthetist demonstrates a reactive habit of action that is based on a preoperative plan, one that is deterministically implemented and in which relevant factual knowledge of drugs is not fully exploited. Furthermore, available patient information provides only a minor basis for regulation of the patient, as if the patient and the information concerning him or her is not related. Some might describe this profile as "cookbook anesthesia" or "anesthesia by numbers."

Based on studies of anesthetists working in their clinical surroundings, Klemola suggests that attempts to improve education and practice should be based on evidence from the real world of anesthetic practice. Learning how to deal with crises through drills with simulators are of practical use, but the educational focus, Klemola (2000) states, should be on developing the intellectual skills of **anticipation** and **making sense of events**, both of which are best learned during clinical work. We suggest that anesthesia training programs must foster an interpretive mindset, one that views as unique both the patient and the patient's response to anesthesia.

As already discussed (see "Individual responsibility within an organization" in Chapter 2), there are other mindsets or mental attitudes that anesthetists should possess if they are to successfully prevent or manage complications during anesthesia, including preparation for the unexpected, early recognition of complications, and an attitude and approach that favor problem-solving, that is, analytical thinking (Klein 1990). Preparation includes a thorough history and physical examination of the patient so as to detect any conditions that may affect anesthesia or that anesthesia may affect. More important, preparation reflects a mental state, one of preparedness or anticipation, that plays a major part in achieving excellence in many activities including anesthesia (Reason 2004). The anesthetist who practices preparedness demonstrates several important characteristics (Reason 2004):

- Accepts that errors can and will occur.
- Assesses the local factors that can cause errors—Reason's "bad stuff" (Reason 2004)—before embarking upon a course of action.
- Has contingency plans ready to deal with anticipated problems.
- Is prepared to seek more qualified assistance.
- Does not let professional courtesy get in the way of checking colleagues' knowledge and experience, particularly when they are strangers (e.g., see Case 6.1).
- Appreciates that the path to adverse incidents is paved with false assumptions.

Reason provides some general guidelines that are applicable to the training of veterinary anesthetists, especially training in error prevention (Reason 1990):

- Training should teach and support an active exploratory approach in which trainees are encouraged to develop their own mental models of the system that they work in, and to use "risky" strategies to investigate and experiment with untaught aspects of the system. This approach recognizes that effective error management is not possible when training is structured according to a set of programmed learning principles, ones that the trainee must follow without question.
- The trainee should have the opportunity to make errors and recover from them. Errors must be viewed as opportunities for learning and discovery so that the trainee overcomes the tendency to view errors as signs of stupidity, lack of intellect, or incompetence. The strategies for dealing with errors have to be both taught and discovered.
- Error training must be introduced at an appropriate phase of training. Introducing it at the beginning of a training program when a trainee is struggling to consciously learn every aspect of a system, may overwhelm the trainee and be counterproductive. Error training may be better introduced at the middle phase of training.

The use of simulators

In-clinic training and experience is crucial, but simulators can be a part of the training process, especially for teaching technical skills such as intubation, intravenous catheterization, epidural or spinal techniques, cardiopulmonary resuscitation (CPR), and teaching strategies for problem-solving. Simulators have also been developed for teaching and improving anesthetists' non-technical skills, such as reactions in a stressful setting, learning, attitudes, behavior, teamwork, and communication skills. High fidelity simulators, those that simulate the real patient, have been developed for use in veterinary medicine, especially emergency medicine (Fletcher *et al.* 2012). Students exposed to this type of training commented that the simulations allowed them to practice communication and teamwork skills better than paper-based, problem-oriented learning opportunities and lectures (Fletcher *et al.* 2012). This is all to the good and complements the essential hands-on clinical training.

Morbidity and mortality rounds (M&Ms)

Processes used to identify errors and near misses, such as morbidity and mortality rounds, should be used as positive, non-threatening educational opportunities to further the organization's patient safety effort (see "Focus groups: morbidity and mortality rounds (M&Ms)" in Chapter 3). They should be used to evaluate the anesthetist's attitude toward errors, and his or her problem-solving skills. In writing about debiasing strategies, Croskerry states that morbidity and mortality rounds "may be a good opportunity for…learning, provided they are carefully and thoughtfully moderated. These rounds tend to inevitably remove the present case from its context and to make it unduly salient in attendees' minds, which may hinder rather than improve future judgment" (Croskerry *et al.* 2013). It is not only the context that may be removed from the discussion, but also the current state of the caregiver at the time of the incident. These are important shortcomings that can be overcome by an effective moderator, one who is knowledgeable about anesthetic processes, able to lead group discussions so that all participants are heard, and do so in a non-judgmental manner. The moderator also must be sensitive to emotional issues that may come to the fore during a case discussion, and be able to recognize and work through individual and group cognitive processes that may make it difficult to get to the root causes of the case under discussion.

Specific strategies for error prevention

Developing a safety culture

Although "safety culture" can be a somewhat nebulous concept, it can be defined as the ideals and beliefs held by an organization toward risk and accidents (safety) and how they influence the thinking and actions of people within the organization. The essence of a safety culture is multifaceted, but revolves around three key concepts:

1 The people performing frontline tasks (those where error most commonly manifests and has impact, such as veterinarians, nurses, and techs on the hospital floor) feel comfortable reporting safety issues to those in charge, specifically to their bosses and upper management.
2 A system is in place to appropriately analyze these reports and management is willing to examine every aspect of the organization and its systems in order to find latent factors or causes of errors.
3 There is a desire and determination to change the organization in order to improve safety.

To achieve a safety culture a number of subcultures need to be developed (Reason 2000); a safety culture needs to be open, just, informed, and flexible, and needs to encourage reporting, learning, and resilience.

An open subculture

Openness means that staff feel comfortable discussing safety incidents and issues during normal working situations rather than only after an incident has occurred or only during a formal investigation. To be successful, openness must extend from the upper echelons of management down to the frontline workers. Senior staff members play vital roles in developing an open work environment because the behavior of those in positions of authority influences the behavior of others. More specifically, for team members to be open about safety issues and "their errors and mistakes" means that

team leaders must be open about their errors and mistakes. Including errors and safety issues in routine clinical discussions brings the subject out into the open—makes it transparent—and demonstrates that "fallibility" is not something to hide. In this way error and safety become a subject for broad discussion, not just for discussions behind closed doors, a management approach that excludes those on the frontline where the errors and accidents occur. Openness keeps safety at the forefront of the organization. Openness also includes transparency and feedback. Staff should know what will happen if and when they report an error and they should be kept informed of where their report is in the analysis process.

Openness does not develop overnight; it is an ongoing process that requires establishing trust and trusted lines of communication between all members of the frontline team, senior staff, and members of management. Although often easier said than done it is a goal worth striving for. To ensure continued development, openness itself needs to be assessed. Face-to-face discussions, surveys, formal interviews, and focus groups can be used to assess the current openness "climate" as viewed by frontline workers, and their current attitudes and concerns about raising safety issues.

A just subculture

When an error occurs, what is the organization's reaction? Is it to focus on discovering who was responsible and punishing or disciplining that person or persons? Or is the organization more lenient and ensures that the people who made the error are given additional training? In either case the focus is on the individual as the root cause of the error, an approach that is often unfair, inappropriate, and counterproductive to achieving a just culture.

When an incident occurs, a "just culture" focuses on the many factors that are responsible, not on who is responsible. It's an organizational culture that does not look for "the culprit," but uses processes that strive to ensure the same error does not occur in the future. A just culture's central tenet is to treat staff fairly and understand that any member of staff at any level of the organization can be involved in a safety incident. The response of a just organization will be to support the individual(s) involved in an incident. This support is intended to help them deal with the consequences of major incidents, to listen to their concerns, and provide an empathetic response while working with them to try to avoid similar problems occurring in the future (see "Analysis of the person(s) at the sharp end: accountability" in Chapter 3, and Figure 3.5).

Superficially this approach may not appear to achieve justice. If someone has done something wrong, that is, made an error, then they should be punished otherwise where is the accountability? As pointed out previously, this approach tends to treat errors as moral issues and is based on the assumption that bad things happen to bad people—the just world hypothesis (Reason 2000). But in Chapters 4 through 7 we have seen how technically competent, knowledgeable, and caring people, good veterinarians and technicians, made errors; disciplining those individuals at the time would not have prevented errors from being made by them or others in the future. Rather, sanctions and punishments breed fear and reduce the likelihood of an individual disclosing and reporting an error, thus driving errors underground.

Accountability should mean encouraging people to be accountable for reporting an incident, instilling in them the importance of sharing their experiences, views, and personal expertise. Accountability means encouraging all members of a team to actively engage in thinking about safety and what can be done about problems that arise and who should be accountable for implementing changes and assessing their effectiveness. This can be considered as forward looking accountability (Dekker 2012).

It is important to recognize that this is not a no-blame culture. An organization should attempt to identify and separate safety incidents involving error (where the events evolved adversely despite the best of intentions) from incidents where staff are deliberately negligent, willfully reckless, or where behavior is not of a required standard. In the latter case not taking action can be seen as unjust and it certainly is a failure of management.

A reporting subculture

In the absence of frequent bad outcomes, knowledge of where the edge lies in regards to safety can only come from persuading those at the human-system interface to report errors (Reason 2000). As discussed in Chapter 3, reporting safety incidents is a powerful tool for gaining information that allows safety improvement strategies to target specific causes of error. Having an open and just culture is fundamental to developing a culture that favors reporting incidents.

However, in and of itself this is insufficient for developing a high rate of reporting in an organization. First and foremost staff must be aware that they are able to report, that there is a reporting system, and that they should use it. Then they must be made aware of what should be reported, how data will be recorded, and how these data will be used. Ensuring that all staff have ready and easy access to the system is also important. Staff need to have confidence that reports will be read and analyzed appropriately, and that they will receive constructive feedback.

A learning subculture

A learning culture means that an organization is able to learn from its errors and that it makes changes in order to reduce the chances of similar errors happening again. This requires the organization as a whole to commit to learning from the incidents that are reported and remembers them over time—keeps them in institutional memory.

An informed subculture

In order to be informed the organization needs to collect and analyze relevant data, and actively distribute to the entire staff the safety information generated from the data. This requires a formal system for distributing safety information. An informed organization also recognizes the importance of prospectively assessing risk, specifically examining and identifying risks in clinical processes before they materialize as incidents.

Flexibility and resilience subcultures

Safety cultures do not come passively into being; they require commitment and effort. They evolve reactively in response to incidents, but more importantly they evolve proactively in response to risk assessment and outside influences. They develop resilience, which is the intrinsic ability of a system to adjust its functioning in response to changes in circumstances so that it can continue to function successfully, even after an adverse incident, or in the presence of continuous stress; that is, the organization is constantly engineering and remolding in the face of new demands. To do this the organization and people within it must be flexible and possess the ability and willingness to continually redesign and manipulate processes where risk is identified. And both must ensure that adequate control measures and barriers are in place.

Minimizing distractions

Distractions are interruptions that are frequently encountered within most healthcare settings, and anesthesia is no exception. Distractions are common causes of broken concentration and in the very least can lead to stress (see "Distractions and stress" in Chapter 2), but at worst can readily lead to error and patient safety incidents. Most often distractions are ordinary events that occur at an inappropriate time. In a busy practice or operating room environment, machines beeping and alarming, phones and pagers ringing and pinging, case discussions, and conversations about the weekend are all commonplace. This is especially pertinent in a teaching hospital where the presence of students and teaching requirements of staff can often lead to impromptu seminars and in-depth explanations. Managing distractions is a key professional skill that is part of the tacit knowledge of anesthesia (Campbell *et al.* 2012).

Most often this hubbub of noise and activity causes little problem and can be tuned out. But there are particular times in various medical processes and procedures that require more concentration than others, when multiple tasks are being performed simultaneously or in rapid succession, during which distractions can have serious consequences.

In a recent study of distractions (Campbell *et al.* 2012) during 30 anesthetics that spanned 30 hours of observation time, 424 distracting events (about one distraction every 4–5 minutes) were observed; distractions in the recovery period occurred most commonly, occurring at about one distraction every 2 minutes. Most of the distractions came from team members and colleagues, while smaller proportions were associated with equipment, workspace, and noise. More specifically, distractions included unrelated conversations, paperwork, being asked questions unrelated to the case, inappropriately timed procedures (including the World Health Organization's Surgical Safety Checklist), overcrowding and space limitations in the workspace, forgotten equipment and drugs, inappropriately set alarms, broken or unchecked equipment, and mobile phones and pagers (Campbell *et al.* 2012). Although a majority of the distractions were of little or no consequence for patients, 92 were judged to have a direct negative effect on anesthetic management. Interestingly, 14 events had positive effects in that they facilitated the procedure or patient safety (Campbell *et al.* 2012). Negative effects included deterioration in a patient's physiological variables, having to repeat procedures, delays in procedures, and periods when the patient was left unattended. This study clearly shows that distractions are common in anesthetic practice and pose a real and significant threat to patient safety. Some distractions, however, are sometimes less obvious and more difficult to observe. Feeling uncomfortable, pain, hunger, being too cold, too hot, unwell, and various emotional states, all can act as distractions and affect our cognitive abilities.

One simple way to help manage distractions is to develop "quiet times," a strategy that has its analogy in aviation, specifically the **sterile cockpit** rule that prohibits non-essential activities during critical phases of flight, especially takeoff and landing, phases analogous to induction of, and emergence from, anesthesia (Broom *et al.* 2011). These are timeouts or pauses at key points of a process, or when multiple tasks are being performed simultaneously. Key points in the process of anesthesia include not only induction of anesthesia, the start of the procedure whatever it may be, and recovery, but also moving/transporting patients, crises, and patient handoffs. Distraction during any one of these phases in the process likely will lead to safety critical steps being missed or vital information concerning a patient not being passed on in an appropriate fashion.

Cognitive forcing: general and specific techniques

Just as some pieces of equipment have design features that prevent their incorrect use (forcing functions), so too are there cognitive forcing strategies. These are specific debiasing techniques or strategies that attempt to minimize influences of irrational decision preferences by introducing self-monitoring into decision-making processes (Croskerry 2003; Stiegler & Ruskin 2012; Stiegler & Tung 2014). Croskerry proposes teaching both generic and specific **cognitive forcing strategies** in clinical decision-making (Croskerry 2003). An example of a generic approach is to teach that one should conduct a secondary search or survey once a positive finding has been made. In other words, once the most spectacular injury has been identified and attended to, a search for a less obvious injury or condition should be made (see Case 6.1). As has been stated in emergency medicine, "the most commonly missed injury in the emergency room is the second" (Stiegler & Tung 2014).

Croskerry has also identified steps to help trainees develop these strategies (Croskerry 2003). First, meta-cognition as a tool, not a theory, should be taught in which the trainee learns the process of thinking about thinking. In practice this requires that the trainee learns to step back from the immediate situation and consider or reflect upon his or her thought processes in the given setting and circumstances, whatever they may be (Croskerry 2003). Are there biases at play in the decision-making process? If so, what are they? The second step is to consider the cognitive errors likely to be made within the given situation, such as an anchoring bias, error of omission, or premature closure (see "Pattern matching and biases" in Chapter 2, and Table 2.3). The third step requires that the trainee imagine the scenario in which a given cognitive error is likely to occur. For example, if an anesthetist is managing emergency anesthesia of a small dog that has been attacked by a larger dog, what biases might be influencing the anesthetist's decision-making in managing this patient? Might a bias or several biases be obscuring his or her diagnostic and management strategy? If so, what would the cognitive error look like? What cognitive forcing strategy should the clinician select?

Anesthesia as a process can be stressful for the anesthetist, and stress can degrade cognitive processes thus fostering the making of errors (see "Distractions and stress" in Chapter 2). An important aspect of training is to teach coping skills that will assist a trainee to overcome stress-induced error-generating tendencies, such as coning of attention and reversion under stress, and start exercising executive-level problem-solving and decision-making skills, that is, the analytical mode of cognition. This can be achieved in part by teaching and reinforcing the fundamentals of anesthesia, such as those techniques that loosen coupling among critical physiological components/systems. Some are very simple techniques and safeguards, including: preoxygenating patients, especially critical patients, prior to induction; assuring that each patient has a patent airway and that the patient is breathing spontaneously if not being mechanically ventilated; rehydrating dehydrated patients prior to anesthesia and maintaining adequate hydration during anesthesia so as to support perfusion of vital organs; keeping patients warm during and after anesthesia; and providing adequate analgesia intra- and post-operatively so as to reduce pain-induced patient stress thus facilitating healing.

Cognitive forcing strategies and the Rule of Three

Stiegler presents four decision-making tools, three to help guide diagnostic and therapeutic intervention, and one to facilitate risk assessment (Stiegler & Ruskin 2012). The **Rule of Three** is one of the tools suggested to help guide clinical reasoning and decision-making (Stiegler & Ruskin 2012). When an anesthetist encounters a problem and the initial and subsequent interventions are unsuccessful, the anesthetist must generate at least three diagnostic possibilities that may explain the cause of the problem before a third intervention is attempted. For example, if a patient is hypotensive and the anesthetist's initial intervention is to lighten the plane of anesthesia, and a few minutes later the second intervention also involves lightening the plane of anesthesia and administering a bolus of fluids, all without correcting the problem, then three other diagnostic possibilities must be considered before a third attempt is made to correct the hypotension (Stiegler & Ruskin 2012). Stiegler points out that the Rule of Three not only forces consideration of alternatives but also prevents specific biases, including premature closure, anchoring, sunk costs, framing, and confirmation bias (see Table 2.3) (Stiegler & Ruskin 2012).

Checklists as error-reducing tools

As already discussed, anesthesia is an inherently complex process. When anesthesia is appropriately performed there are a large number of tasks that must be undertaken before a patient can be anesthetized. Many tasks are performed automatically, at the skill-based level, but in a busy practice environment it is inevitable that a task or item will be missed (omission error). The effect of these lapses may seem insignificant to those involved, perhaps only leading to a delay in the progress of the case or a temporary distraction. But as mentioned previously, in an emergent situation such lapses may delay care of the patient, and some steps, of course, are fundamental to anesthesia management, and failure to perform them could have major consequences for patient safety. Checklists are a means for minimizing errors of omission and are now commonplace in most complex workplaces and professions (for a more complete history of checklists see Appendix E).

The role of a checklist is to ensure that the person(s) performing a task or involved in a process will not need to rely on memory. In essence it helps ensure that tasks are performed and by the appropriate time in the process. It is important to recognize that a checklist is not a step-by-step guide or algorithm for performing a task. Although these tools can be useful for novices and inexperienced staff, they tend to be used less and considered less helpful by more experienced members, who tend to ignore steps or perform multiple tasks at the same time. The problem here, of course, is that missing one step can lead to subsequent steps being missed, any one of which might be a safety-critical step, one that if omitted will lead to a near miss or worse a harmful incident.

The essence of a checklist is to include tasks or actions critical to the smooth running and performance of a process; as such it forms the basis of procedural standardization. Tasks on a checklist should be chosen according to their relative importance in terms of whether failing to perform a task or action (at all or appropriately) will compromise safety, and what the potential is for that task being overlooked (i.e., likely not to be checked by some other mechanism). The order of the checklist will typically be that in which the tasks or actions are normally performed. The performance of a checklist signifies the end of one phase of a process and indicates that all the vital and relevant tasks have been completed in order to move safely to the next phase.

A checklist can be used in two ways: (1) the **call-do-response** (or do-list), and (2) the **challenge-response** (Degani & Wiener 1993). Using the call-do-response method the checklist items are called out prospectively, each acting as a prompt to perform the specific task. Each task or action is then performed and then confirmed before moving onto the next step. In the challenge-response method the tasks are performed according to memory and the checklist is used retrospectively to ensure that each task or action has been performed. The challenge-response method is generally considered more suitable for most situations as it allows more flexibility in the process and is an acknowledgment that tasks may not be performed in the order designated by the checklist.

Checklist design requires consideration of content, format, and timing; as such checklists should (Degani & Wiener 1993):

- Provide a standard foundation for verifying that a process is or has been carried out in a thorough and appropriate fashion in an attempt to defeat any impairment to a team's psychological and physical condition.

- Provide a sequential framework to tasks.
- Allow mutual supervision (cross-checking) among team members.
- Identify and assign the duties of each team member in order to facilitate optimum team coordination as well as logical distribution of workload.
- Enhance a team approach through effective communication ensuring that each team member at each phase is kept in the loop.

Checklists should be tested, and those testing them should have the ability to provide feedback and make suggestions as to alterations and adaptations. Ideally, checklists will then be evaluated and tested in a more formal and scientific fashion. When designing a checklist there are a number of key components that must be considered (Nagano 1975):

- Checklists should have a clear objective.
- Checklists should be practicable.
- Every item on the checklist should be a safety-critical step that is at risk of being missed and that inclusion on the checklist can help rectify.
- Checklist items should be based on sound evidence or be indisputable in terms of their importance to the process.
- Checklists should be designed to fit in at natural breaks in workflow "pause points" so as not to disrupt the normal process.
- Checklists should be clear and precise, containing simple, brief items.
- Checklists should be easy to perform; using simple exact language and a sentence structure designed to be read aloud.
- Checklists should have a logical and linear progression.
- Checklists should have fewer than 8–10 items per pause point.
- Checklists should encourage communication of critical information to team members and facilitate teamwork. (As Leape stated, "[checklists are] a tool for ensuring that team communication happens" (Leape 2014)).
- Checklists must be well grounded within the "present day" operational environment so that the team will have a sound realization of their importance, and not regard them as a nuisance or antiquated task.

Checklists in medicine

Checklists have been around in medicine for some time in one form or another, although some formats are barely recognizable as checklists. Most anesthetists are familiar with an anesthetic machine checklist and, in a way, filling in an anesthetic chart is a continually cycling checklist of a patient's vital signs. However, the checklist as a safety tool in medicine was not really heralded until 2004 when a critical care team led by Peter Pronovost developed a set of clinical guidelines and accompanying checklist for reducing central line infections (Berenholtz *et al.* 2004), guidelines that were validated in 2006 (Pronovost *et al.* 2006).

It was a simple, evidence-based, pragmatic, and commonsense guideline consisting of six major steps (Berenholtz *et al.* 2004): (1) hand washing; (2) sterilization of the insertion site; (3) draping the entire patient; (4) using sterile gloves, a mask, hat, and gown; (5) maintaining a sterile field; and (6) applying a sterile dressing to the insertion site. Before the introduction of the checklist, doctors only followed the evidence-based guidelines in 62% of central catheter insertions; as a result, catheter-related infections occurred at a rate of 11.3 per 1000 catheter days. Astonishingly, after the checklist was introduced the rate decreased to 0 infections per 1000 catheter days. It was estimated that 43 catheter-related infections had been avoided and that eight lives had been saved with the added bonus of potentially saving almost US$2,000,000 in additional healthcare costs over a year (Berenholtz *et al.* 2004).

This checklist was not created in isolation as no checklist in and of itself will guarantee safety. Four other separate and concurrent interventions were implemented with the central line checklist:

1 ICU staff were educated about the importance of catheter site infections and evidence-based guidelines.
2 A "catheter insertion cart" was created that contained all the equipment needed to perform catheterization according to the guidelines.
3 As part of the daily ICU rounds clinicians were asked whether catheters could be removed, thus removing a source of infection when it was no longer vital to patient care.
4 Nurses were empowered to challenge doctors and stop the catheter being inserted if a violation of the checklist was observed.

The most heralded and well-publicized of all healthcare checklists is the World Health Organization's Safe Surgical Checklist (Haynes *et al.* 2009; Safe Surgery Saves Lives Programme Team 2009). A team of multidisciplinary experts led by Dr Atul Gawande were tasked

---

Box 8.2 Ten universal factors regarding surgical safety (Safe Surgery Saves Lives Programme Team 2009).

1 Correct patient at the correct site	6 Minimizing risk of surgical site infection
2 Provision of safe anesthesia	7 Preventing retention of swabs and instruments
3 Management of airway problems	8 Accurate identification of specimens
4 Management of hemorrhage	9 Effective communication within the surgical team
5 Avoiding known allergies	10 Routine surveillance of surgical outcomes

---

with developing interventions that could improve safety for surgical patients. (The full story behind this checklist is reported by Atul Gawande in his book *The Checklist Manifesto*, Profile Books, 2010.) Based upon available evidence and expert opinion, 10 universal factors regarding surgical safety were recognized (Safe Surgery Saves Lives Programme Team 2009) (Box 8.2).

A 19-item checklist was designed to incorporate these factors (Weiser *et al.* 2010). Breaks in workflow were recognized as: the point immediately prior to induction; the point immediately before first incision; and the point at which the patient leaves the operating room and is recovered from anesthesia. Elements of the checklist were assigned to the appropriate workflow time points and the Safe Surgical Checklist was born.

During initial testing the effect of the checklist was impressive (Weiser *et al.* 2010). Eight hospitals from different countries and socioeconomic settings recorded data for 30-day survival and complications following surgery before and after implementation of the checklist. Almost 8000 surgical procedures were enrolled; fatalities dropped from 1.5% to 0.8% and complications from 11% to 7%. It is not clear which elements of the checklist were responsible for these dramatic effects, but it appeared to be more than the sum of its parts. Some effects were obvious, such as ensuring that antibiotics were administered at the critical time; however, others were intangible, such as the effect of improving teamwork and communication (briefing and debriefing components of the checklist). The effect of checklists on teamwork and communication has subsequently been confirmed as an important factor in improving patient safety (Russ *et al.* 2013).

Ongoing research into the effects of checklists has been mixed. Most often the outcomes are improved, as with the World Health Organization's Surgical Checklist (Haynes *et al.* 2009), but other studies have shown little or no significant difference (Gagliardi *et al.* 2014; Urbach *et al.* 2014). Although the degree of their impact is variable, any effect is generally positive, insofar as no checklist has been shown to be detrimental (Thomassen *et al.* 2014; Treadwell *et al.* 2014). The reality is that a checklist cannot be universally effective; its efficacy will be related to the likelihood that any particular organization or healthcare provider will not perform a necessary step in the checklist. In Leape's words, "it is not the act of ticking off a checklist that reduces complications, but performance of the actions it calls for" (Leape 2014). The efficacy of a checklist also depends on the safety culture and other safety mechanisms at play in any particular organization.

Leape has presented several reasons why checklists can fail to show significant improvements (Leape 2014). Firstly, changing practice is difficult and cannot be achieved solely by ticking boxes. Successfully changing a system and modifying human behavior and interactions is complex. To make these changes requires demonstrating the need for change, engaging leaders and management in the change process, collecting adequate data, and developing teamwork so that everyone feels involved, respected, and accountable (Vogus & Hilligoss 2015).

Secondly, the checklist has to be used properly. There are individuals who will resist using the checklist and when these individuals are in positions of power and authority the checklist will fail; it will not be used as intended, or, when the authority figure is present, the checklist will be used in a cursory or rushed manner. Alternatively, some hospitals may lack the resources or expertise to effectively implement a checklist and as a result team members may be less experienced and inadequately trained.

Thirdly, checklists are not a quick fix. Full implementation takes time and effort, and effects may not be seen immediately. Although each of the individual checks may seem straightforward, appropriately performing a checklist requires training and practice. Importantly, modifications and adaptations may also be required to make the checklist "fit" the local system. Where this does not occur, conflict between the checklist and workflow may occur and the checklist will become viewed as a burdensome, tiresome chore that has to be performed but without influencing practice.

There are other reasons why checklists may not be welcomed by all. Some people dislike and fear checklists because they view them as dehumanizing, and clinicians feel that they impinge on their clinical freedom. Often they confuse a checklist with a standard operating procedure or clinical guidelines. They may view checklists as a means by which their work is assessed, of being monitored so that administrators can make sure they are doing their work properly. However, this mindset misses the reasons for a good checklist: it is not meant to dictate the way or how a process is performed or who performs a given task, but rather to ensure vital safety steps are performed. Most often the tasks and actions on a checklist are not disputable, they are common sense or evidence-based and are actions that should always be performed.

Often those opposed to checklists are those who forget that they themselves are capable of making mistakes and may argue, "If checklists contain vital instructions and tasks, then everyone should know that they have to be done anyway, right? So why do we need a checklist?" They may state, "How anyone could get this wrong is beyond me!" They do not understand how they and others can make errors or mistakes. Often these individuals may be experienced, senior colleagues who have forgotten that modern medicine is a team effort and that all team members do not function alike. Or they may be individuals who lack confidence and dislike being questioned about patient management. It should be noted in both circumstances that the checklist benefits the team and the patient; the checklist is not aimed at the individual caregiver.

In conclusion, checklists have a huge potential for improving safety in anesthesia. However, checklists can only be successful when they are well designed, used appropriately and at the correct time, and when they are integrated into a matrix of other safety initiatives (Vogus & Hilligoss 2015).

Where can I utilize checklists in my anesthetic process?

There are numerous times when checklists can be used in most practices to help enhance patient safety during anesthesia. The classic example and probably best known checklist is the FDA's Anesthesia Apparatus Checkout (see Appendix F) of the anesthetic machine and equipment. Although this checklist dates from 1993, it is applicable today because most anesthesia machines in use in veterinary anesthesia, at least in the United States today in private practice, are based on models covered by this checklist. More fundamentally, the checklist is an excellent guide to both the process and what must be considered when checking out anesthesia-related equipment. There are newer and multiple variations of machine checklists in existence today; most are published as either a checklist or as a form that can readily be converted into a checklist. These checklists are designed to be used with modern, hi-tech anesthetic machines for use with human patients and some of the items to be checked may not be applicable to many veterinary practices. For this reason the Association of Veterinary Anaesthetists (AVA) launched an Anaesthetic Safety Checklist in September, 2014, which may be more applicable globally in veterinary anesthesia (see Appendix G).

There are other checklists that may be used during the peri-anesthetic period, such as the World Health Organization's Safe Surgical Checklist, but it highlights anesthesia in only four specific statements:
- Is the anesthesia machine and medication check complete?
- Is the pulse oximeter on the patient and functioning?
- To anesthetist: Are there any patient-specific concerns?
- To surgeon, anesthetist, and nurse: What are the key concerns for recovery and management of this patient?

These four points, however, do not cover the full spectrum of anesthetic safety-critical tasks that must be performed. The Association of Veterinary Anaesthetists' Anaesthetic Safety Checklist addresses this shortcoming by using the same pause points of pre-induction, pre-procedure and pre-recovery as a means for making a number of anesthesia-specific checks (see Appendix G). However, some other safety-critical information is not included in that checklist, such as the administration of antibiotics.

Checklists can also be utilized in other less routine situations. For example, a difficult airway checklist could be developed for patients at risk of airway obstruction or aspiration at induction. The checklist could consist of the following items in addition to those set out in the AVA Anaesthetic Safety Checklist:
- Suction and swabs.
- Range of endotracheal tube types and sizes.

- Guidewire or stylet +/− insufflation device (a device combining the two can be made by attaching a stiff male dog urinary catheter to a syringe barrel—plunger removed—and attaching a tight-fitting endotracheal tube connector to the other end of the syringe barrel).
- A kit for percutaneous oxygen insufflation (either a percutaneous tracheostomy kit or a wire bore needle attached to a syringe barrel and endotracheal tube connector as above).
- Patient positioned in sternal recumbency without external pressure on the abdomen prior to induction.

Checklists of this nature have far more flexibility and usability than protocol-based anesthetics that dictate every clinical step and decision. These checklists allow a high degree of clinical freedom and judgment and may be more likely to be followed as they allow individuals to manage most aspects of the case such as drug selection while ensuring that basic safety equipment is available. Because these types of checklists are more broad and universal in scope than are protocols, they are more likely to be used in patients that fall outside the target population of a protocol; this is beneficial because there is a tendency to think that when one step of a process is irrelevant to an individual patient then the rest of the protocol is too, when such is not the case.

Checklists in crises

So far we have only considered checklists designed for use during normal circumstances. What about abnormal, crisis, or emergency situations? Do checklists just take time and divert attention away from the truly important focus of the crisis: the patient? After all, crises are often characterized by factors that may conspire to make them very challenging to manage (Runciman & Merry 2005):
- Crises may present with opaque, non-specific signs or symptoms.
- Crises may arise from the interaction of many complex factors.
- The problems may evolve, revealing additional layers of complexity.
- The particular set of circumstances may never have been encountered before.
- Recently introduced processes and equipment may bring new unforeseen problems.
- Skilled assistance may not be available in the necessary time frame.
- Crises may have to be resolved very rapidly if disaster is to be averted.

Can checklists work in these situations and reduce the chance of missing a potentially lifesaving step? The experience of aviation and other high reliability organizations suggests that the answer is a resounding YES!

The ever influential Dr Atul Gawande and colleagues devised a set of checklists to combat 12 of the most frequently occurring operating room crises: air embolism, anaphylaxis, unstable bradycardia, cardiac arrest (asystole/pulseless electrical activity), cardiac arrest (ventricular fibrillation/ventricular tachycardia), failed airway, fire, hemorrhage, hypotension, hypoxia, malignant hyperthermia, and unstable tachycardia (Arriaga *et al.* 2013). These checklists were based upon evidence-based metrics of essential care for each of the crises. These checklists went through multiple iterations and were then tested and refined following small-scale simulations. Subsequently, the group performed larger scale assessments and observed operating room teams in a series of 106 simulated surgical-crisis scenarios (Arriaga *et al.* 2013). Each team was randomly assigned to manage half the scenarios with a set of the crisis checklists, and the remaining scenarios were managed using memory alone. When a checklist was unavailable the failure to perform potentially lifesaving processes was 23%, but this was reduced to 6% when checklists were available.

These checklists were designed to be used when the cause of the crisis is not immediately known, or where the most appropriate intervention should occur but is not immediately obvious. For these situations, Runciman and Merry have described why algorithms and checklists can be invaluable (Runciman & Merry 2005). The task of the anesthesiologist during a crisis is a challenging one; first they need to confirm that a crisis is actually occurring; secondly they should attempt to diagnose the cause of the crisis; thirdly they need to make appropriate interventions in order to resolve the crisis; and finally they must continue being vigilant and monitor for recurrence of the problem or additional crises. From available data it is clear that crises are not always managed adequately, and the consequences of this inadequacy are sometimes fatal. Checklists can be designed to help overcome these shortcomings. It is important to recognize that in these situations, properly designed checklists are designed to assist analytical modes of problem-solving and not replace them; they are prompts to ensure a thorough approach and not necessarily algorithms to follow without question.

Mnemonics

A mnemonic is a device that may use a pattern of letters, words, a song, ideas, or associations to aid memory. The following mnemonics have been developed for use in anesthesia as means to assist anesthetists avoid making errors by moving them from intuitive thinking to analytical thinking, that is, to move from rule-based cognitive processing to knowledge-based analytical cognitive processing (see Figure 6.5). These mnemonics also help confront biases that may be affecting cognitive processes, or serve as mental checklists to help an anesthetist quickly and effectively rule out a wide range of potentially lethal problems that can occur during emergent situations in anesthesia.

The 3-P mnemonic

The 3-P mnemonic (Stiegler & Ruskin 2012) is a simple tool by which the anesthetist **Perceives** that the clinical situation has changed, **Processes** this information and determines a course of action to achieve a desired outcome, and then **Performs** the needed action(s). This, of course, is a closed loop, one in which the anesthetist is brought back to the beginning to perceive if the intervention has in fact produced the desired effect within an appropriate time frame (Stiegler & Ruskin 2012). If the desired effect has not occurred, then the anesthetist has either misdiagnosed the problem or used an incorrect intervention. According to Stiegler, this tool helps to prevent knowledge-based errors (mistakes) and slips, and forces the anesthetist to re-evaluate the clinical situation rather than continuing to follow an incorrect course of action (Stiegler & Ruskin 2012).

DECIDE

The DECIDE mnemonic and the model it rests on is again meant to move the anesthetist from intuitive thinking to analytical thinking, by forcing him or her to actively consider a problem and pursue a course of action to resolve it (see "Error causation: human factors" in Chapter 2). This model consists of six steps (Stiegler & Ruskin 2012):

D—Detect that something has changed

E—Estimate the need to react to the change

C—Choose a desirable outcome

I—Identify the action(s) needed to achieve the desired outcome

D—Do the necessary action(s)

E—Evaluate the effects of the action(s).

The second item, E, in the above list raises the concept of action limits, those patient-related physiological limits that when exceeded trigger an intervention by the anesthetist. For example, what arterial blood pressure triggers a response by an anesthetist to treat a hypotensive or hypertensive patient? We all have our action limits and use them to guide anesthetic management. A survey of a very small number of diplomates of the American College of Veterinary Anesthesia and Analgesia (ACVAA) indicated that their preferred ranges for selected variables in anesthetized dogs were:

- Mean arterial blood pressure (MAP): range 70 to 120 mmHg
- SpO_2: >94–95%
- $P_E'CO_2$: range 35 to 55 mmHg (the higher value only if the patient's brain is normal)

A more extensive online survey (Ruffato *et al.* 2015) of diplomates of the ACVAA and of the European College of Veterinary Anaesthesia and Analgesia, defined hypotension in dogs undergoing anesthesia and surgery as systolic arterial blood pressures (SAP) <87 ± 8 mmHg, while in dogs undergoing anesthesia for diagnostic procedures it was defined as a SAP of <87 ± 6 mmHg; mean arterial pressure (MAP) defining hypotension for both types of patients was <62 ± 4 mmHg. The averages of the pressures that prompted treatment of canine surgical patients were a SAP of 85 ± 13 mmHg or a MAP of 61 ± 4 mmHg; for patients undergoing diagnostic procedures a SAP of 84 ± 11 mmHg or a MAP of 63 ± 8 mmHg triggered treatment (Ruffato *et al.* 2015).

The following is not meant to belittle action limits, but it must be kept in mind that these thresholds are for one species and may not be applicable to other species (they may also be inappropriate for subpopulations of a species such as neonatal or pediatric patients). For example, a $P_E'CO_2$ of 55 mmHg in a bird would be considered too high; such a value has been associated with cardiac arrhythmias in birds anesthetized with halothane (Naganobu *et al.* 2001).

It is also important to consider that threshold-based guidelines are not the only way of triggering interventions. When anesthetists see an anesthetized animal's blood pressure decrease suddenly from a MAP of 100 mmHg to 70 mmHg, they are obviously unlikely to delay intervention until the ~60 mmHg threshold is reached. In fact proactive management is expected. Another example where action limits can

fail is heart rate. A heart rate of 40 beats per minute in a dog premedicated with a combination of acepromazine and an opioid probably should be treated, but if the dog was premedicated with a combination of dexmedetomidine and an opioid, then the bradycardia is expected and is considered a normal response to the dexmedetomidine. Administering an anticholinergic in the first case would be appropriate, but it could result in unacceptable hypertension in the latter case. Assessment of blood pressure in either case would be required in order to make an informed decision on treating the bradycardia or not.

So these parameters we measure, and upon which we base our decision-making, need to be considered within the context of the individual patient. But the principle of action limits is valid across species as long as the action limit is considered within an analytical framework.

FORDEC

Another mnemonic, one borrowed from the airline industry, that works well as a mental checklist in time-sensitive situations requiring urgent decision-making, is FORDEC (Hubler *et al.* 2014):

F—Facts: collection of all relevant facts

O—Options: collection of alternative actions

R—Risks: considering F and O, consider the chances of success for each action

D—Decision: the action most likely to succeed is chosen, with possible backup plans

E—Execute: the chosen action is carried out

C—Check: compare the action and success with the expected result

PAVE

When developing and executing an anesthetic protocol, anesthetists must consider possible risks to the patient. To do so Stiegler presents another mnemonic, one originally developed by the US Federal Aviation Administration. This mnemonic was based on Pilot, Aircraft, Environment, and External Pressure—**PAVE** (Stiegler & Ruskin 2012). Stiegler has modified the mnemonic for use by anesthetists:

P—Patient: illness or reason it is undergoing anesthesia and comorbidities.

A—Anesthetist: training and skills, recent experience, fatigue.

V—EnVironment: where the procedure will be performed, available equipment and supplies, and who will be available to help if a problem arises.

E—External pressures: production pressure, pressure from the owner or surgeon.

COVER ABCD and A SWIFT CHECK

The Australian Incident Monitoring Study (AIMS) developed mnemonics—COVER ABCD and A SWIFT CHECK—to help guide problem-solving when a case is not progressing as planned; these mental tools are meant to help move thinking from the intuitive rule-based mode to the analytical level, so as to quickly and effectively rule out a wide range of potentially lethal problems (Runciman & Merry 2005; Runciman *et al.* 1993, 2005). Both have been adapted for use in veterinary anesthesia at University Queen's Veterinary School Hospital, University of Cambridge. This adapted 'COVERED' mnemonic is shown in Table 8.2.

The 'A SWIFT CHECK' mnemonic has been adapted for use at the Queen's Veterinary Hospital, and is a secondary diagnostic strategy that aims to highlight the most common and likely causes of anesthetic crises (Table 8.3). These adaptations have been made because some of the original elements in the Australian Incident Monitoring Study mnemonics are not directly applicable to veterinary practice as some involve tasks or actions that are not valid or are unavailable to veterinary patients. Neither of the mnemonics is supposed to be memorized, but they should be immediately available in any facility where an anesthetized patient may be managed. At the end of each checklist is Runciman's cautionary message: "If the problem has not been solved, direct the available resources to its solution. Get skilled and experienced help. Work from first principles" (Runciman *et al.* 2005).

To aid ready access to these mnemonics, each final year student and staff member rotating through the

Table 8.2 A mnemonic to help move problem-solving to the analytical level of thinking. This mnemonic was developed by Dr M. McMillan and is used at the University Queen's Veterinary School Hospital, University of Cambridge, whenever there is a concern about the safety of an anesthetized patient.

	Communicate	Communicate concerns with surgeon. Alert team. Raise alarm.
C	**Circulation**	Check the patient's pulse rate, character, and rhythm to gain an impression of the adequacy of their circulatory status. Does CPR need to be instigated?
	Color	Check the patient's mucous membrane colour. Signs of cyanosis (pulse oximetry is recommended as visual cyanosis is a late sign)? Pallor? Toxemia/sepsis/hypercarbia?
O	**Oxygen**	Check anesthetic machine flowmeter. Ensure administering 100% O_2. If using oxygen concentrator, ensure concentrator appears to be working (ideally check with an oxygen analyzer)
V	**Ventilation**	Is patient breathing spontaneously? Is reservoir bag moving? Hand ventilate patient's lungs. Assess breathing system and airway patency, thoracic wall motion, thoracic compliance. If using a capnograph is there a good trace?
E	**ET tube**	Check the ET tube for kinks/leaks/obstructions. Is the ET tube overlong (endobronchial intubation)?
R	**Review**	Review all monitors and equipment
	Evaluation	Cross-reference. Does everything fit and is everything in agreement? Does anything stand out?
E	**Elimination**	Check the patient's depth of anesthesia. Check vaporizer settings and level of agent. Consider turning off vaporizer. Administer 100% O_2. If using a circle breathing system consider changing breathing system or disconnecting patient and using O_2 flush
D	**Drugs**	Could problem be due to an adverse effect of a drug? Overdose? Rate of administration?

Modified for use in veterinary anesthesia from: Runciman, W.B., *et al.* (2005) Crisis management during anaesthesia: the development of an anaesthetic crisis management manual. *Quality & Safety in Health Care* **14**:e1 (http://www.qshc.com/cgi/content/full/14/3/e1). With permission of the publisher.

Table 8.3 A mnemonic and secondary diagnostic algorithm that can be used to highlight all of the most common and likely causes of crises encountered during anesthesia. It is meant to help move problem-solving to the analytical level of thinking. Developed by Dr M. McMillan, it is used at Cambridge University Queen's Veterinary School Hospital.

	Check	Signs	Causes
A	**Awakening**	Tachycardia, apnea, hyperventilation, hypertension, movement, increased muscle tone	Failure of anesthetic administration (disconnection, failed IV, delivery device), resistant patient
	Abdomen	Mixed cardiovascular and respiratory effects—tachycardia & hypotension, hypoventilation & hypoxemia	Gastric or intestinal dilatation, torsion of viscus, bladder distension
	Anaphylaxis	Hypotension, tachycardia, bronchospasm, urticaria	Any drugs (antibiotics), transfused blood products, human albumin
S	**Surgery**	Mixed	Vagal stimulation, caval compression, hemorrhage, pain, release of vasoactive substances
W	**Weight**	Mixed—often hypotension and ventilation/oxygenation issues	Diaphragmatic splinting, caval compression, reduced functional residual capacity (FRC)
I	**Inflammation**	Hypotension, massive vasodilation	Sepsis/systemic inflammatory response syndrome (SIRS)
	IV access	Failure to respond as expected to IV drug administration	Cannula no longer patent (clot, kink), dislodged
F	**Fluids**	Mixed	Fluid overload, electrolyte disturbance
T	**Trauma**	Mixed	Pulmonary or cardiac contusions, pneumothorax, ruptured bladder, occult hemorrhage
	Temperature	Hypothermia—bradycardia, hypotension, low respiratory rate and hypocapnia, increased depth of anesthesia	Failure of heating device
		Hyperthermia—tachycardia, hypertension, tachypnea, decreased depth of anesthesia	Drugs, inhalants, heating device
	Transfusion	Tachycardia, hypotension, hypoxemia, urticaria, bronchoconstriction	Transfusion reaction to blood products or albumin
C	**Cardiac**	Arrhythmia, hypotension, poor pulse quality	Occult cardiac disease, myocardial or valvular dysfunction
H	**Hypoglycemia**	Bradycardia, hypotension, hypothermia, increased depth of anesthesia	Liver dysfunction, insulin, paraneoplastic
E	**Embolus**	Hypotension, hypocapnia, arrhythmia	Air, fat, thrombus
	Endocrine	Mixed	Thyroid, adrenals, diabetes
C	**Ca²⁺**	Hypercalcemia—arrhythmia Hypocalcaemia—muscle weakness, tachycardia, arrhythmia	Renal, hyperparathyroidism, toxicity, paraneoplastic Acidosis, toxicity, inflammatory disease, pregnancy
K	**K⁺**	Hyperkalemia—bradycardia, arrhythmia	Acute kidney injury, urethral obstruction, urinary tract rupture, hypoadrenocorticism, cell lysis, over-administration of KCl
		Hypokalaemia—muscle weakness, tachycardia, arrhythmia	Inappetance, fluid therapy, renal losses, GI losses

Modified for use in veterinary anesthesia from: Runciman, W.B., *et al.* (2005) Crisis management during anaesthesia: the development of an anaesthetic crisis management manual. *Quality & Safety in Health Care* **14**:e1 (http://www.qshc.com/cgi/content/full/14/3/e1). With permission of the publisher.

anesthesia service at the Queen's Veterinary School Hospital, is given a pocket-sized handbook with the COVERED mnemonic and A SWIFT CHECK checklist, along with a list of critical clinical conditions that may be encountered during anesthesia (including possible causes and management strategies; see Appendix H), a number of approaches for anesthesia in various species, and a formulary. The mnemonic and checklist are intended to be used when initial intuitive and rule-based problem-solving has failed. An initial subjective impression is that students and inexperienced staff members (residents and interns), when they have this checklist, feel better equipped and able to deal with crises that occur during anesthesia clinics. Of course staff and students are not expected to deal with problems alone, unsupervised, or that are beyond their capabilities. It does mean that during the time from when help has been requested and it arrives the checklist will have been followed and the crisis will more likely be under control.

Structured communication: a beginning, middle, and an end

In clinics we need to communicate all of the time and generally do so in specific ways depending on the situation and the audience. For example, when presenting a case in rounds we generally follow the linear order of history, physical examination, problem list, differential diagnosis, diagnostic tests, and so forth. This structured approach best allows information to be followed and understood by the audience. To demonstrate this point let's imagine trying to communicate information with the following words:

> the information from the understanding of the words think, held about in the structure and a punctuation, but comes the order the sentence is the words.

They make little sense, it's frustrating if not painful to read, and difficult to remember. However, when this information is restructured according to rules of grammar and syntax it suddenly becomes understandable and easily remembered:

> think about a sentence, the information is held in the words but the understanding comes from the structure, the order of the words and the punctuation.

Structure is vital in communication. Information is best passed on in a logical, structured, and familiar format. Using a template can help standardize the manner in which information is transferred, and in critical situations where there is no room for miscommunication, the use of templates improves information transfer.

One of the most recognized information templates in medicine is the SOAP—Subjective, Objective, Assessment, Plan—a method of recording medical notes introduced in 1968 by Dr Lawrence Weed, father of the problem-orientated medical record (POMR); its purpose was and still is to provide an organized means of recording patient data that acts as both a guide and teaching aid for those involved in a patient's care (Weed 1968). The **subjective** component is a narrative description of the patient's condition and the information generally is in the form of unmeasurable evaluations based on the clinician's opinion. The **objective** component documents repeatable, measurable evaluations that can be followed over time to identify patterns and changes; physiological measurements (e.g., heart rate, blood pressure, physical examination findings, bodyweight, pain scales/scores, etc.), and laboratory results (e.g. PCV, total protein, electrolytes, etc.) are classic examples. The **assessment** records the clinician's general appraisal of the situation, which often consists of an evolving problem list, differential/working/actual diagnosis, and evaluation of the progress of the patient. The **plan** consists of the proposed management of the patient, including diagnostic and therapeutic procedures/measures (e.g., medications, laboratory tests, diagnostic imaging, surgery, etc.). Is this the best method for patient hand-offs, a critical and error-prone event, especially during anesthesia? Before answering this question, let's first consider what hand-offs entail.

Hand-offs between anesthetists, or between anesthetists and staff in recovery rooms or intensive care units are performed at times of considerable stress, for example, during an anesthetic or when a patient is recovering from anesthesia. The latter situation can be very challenging and stressful because recovering patients are in a precarious and rapidly changing condition and yet during this time many tasks need to be completed that can distract both the individual transferring the patient and the individual receiving the patient. However, whether during anesthesia or recovery, both situations require transferring large amounts of information that are vital and applicable to the patient's immediate and ongoing care. It is not surprising that communication errors can occur during these hand-offs. So, is there a method for minimizing errors during patient hand-offs?

Other systems have been developed to assist in rapid and accurate transfers of critical information such as patient hand-offs. One such system is SBAR—Situation, Background, Assessment, Recommendation—initially devised by the military, a template perhaps appropriate for patient hand-offs. The following describes the elements as they might occur during the hand-off of a patient from an anesthetist to a recovery room technician:

Situation—the anesthetist gives to the recovery room technician the patient's name and signalment, a brief description of the procedure, and duration of anesthesia.

Background—provides the context that contains a synopsis of the patient's essential clinical information and history, including the patient's problem list (any morbidities or comorbidities), any procedural or anesthetic complications, and any interventions that were made.

Assessment—outlines the patient's current status, including what is now going on with the patient or might be going on. This must include assessments of the patient's airway, breathing, and cardiovascular system, body temperature, fluid balance, and pain status. The assessment should include information on severity and urgency of any problems; likely complications should be outlined.

Recommendation—concisely summarizes ongoing patient management, including what needs to be done with the patient both in terms of monitoring and treatments. Alarm limits and interventions for likely complications should be discussed and set during this period. If the patient should deteriorate, the person to contact should be clearly identified with all necessary contact information (pager number, cell phone number).

The goal of any hand-off is to prevent a break in the flow of patient care provided by caregivers when there is a change in personnel; the hallmark of a successful hand-off is a smooth continuity of patient care from one caregiver to the next (Patterson & Woods 2001). The use of SBAR during hand-offs may facilitate transfer of patient, anesthetic, and surgical information and reduce errors of omission. But this system of verbal communication merely provides a general outline for communications and does not ensure all of the essential clinical information is transmitted effectively. And, even if all information is transmitted, it does not mean the information will be received and recalled, so verbal communications should also be backed up with written documentation presented in the same structure and format (Nagpal *et al.* 2010). A more thorough approach to patient hand-offs has been outlined by Patterson, who described 21 actions and changes in process that can help to reduce communication failure during the hand-off process (Patterson *et al.* 2004):

Improve hand-off update effectiveness

1 Face-to-face verbal update with interactive questioning.
2 Additional update from practitioners other than the one being replaced.
3 Limit interruptions during update.
4 Topics initiated by incoming as well as outgoing personnel.
5 Limit initiation of operator actions during update.
6 Include outgoing team's stance toward changes to plans and contingency plans.
7 Read-back to ensure that information was accurately received.

Improve hand-off update efficiency and effectiveness

8 Outgoing caregiver writes summary before hand-off.
9 Incoming caregiver assesses current status.
10 Update information in the same order every time.
11 Incoming scans historical data before update.
12 Incoming reviews automatically captured changes to sensor-derived data before update.
13 Intermittent monitoring of system status while on call.
14 Outgoing has knowledge of previous shift activities.

Increase access to data

15 Incoming caregiver receives primary access to the most up-to-date information.
16 Incoming receives paperwork that includes handwritten annotations.
17 Unambiguous transfer of responsibility.
18 Make it clear to others who is responsible for which duties at a particular time.
19 Overhear others' updates.

Enable error detection and recovery

20 Outgoing caregiver oversees incoming caregiver's work following update.

Delay transfer of responsibility during critical activities

21 Delay the transfer of responsibility when concerned about status/stability of process.

Incorporating all of these considerations into patient hand-offs should help limit communication breakdowns and ensure that information is passed effectively from caregiver to caregiver thus limiting the opportunities for errors.

Evaluating the process of anesthesia: systems walk

A systems walk can be used to prospectively assess the safety of the anesthetic processes in an organization or practice, and helps to adapt or redesign the processes with patient safety in mind. Many actions that improve safety may also improve efficiency, often with minimal cost in terms of time and money for implementation. Experienced clinicians, nurses, and technicians all develop a degree of error wisdom or foresight that enables them to become effective error spotters. Newer, less experienced staff, on the other hand, have a different set of skills and are useful as they are often more open-minded and, if empowered, may be more likely to challenge pre-existing processes while adding fresh perspectives and new ideas in the assessment process. These varied skills should be harnessed, so when performing a systems walk it is useful to have a mix of staff to utilize the group's "collective error wisdom" and open-mindedness.

In terms of an anesthesia systems walk, the idea would be to plot the steps required to admit, anesthetize, recover, and discharge a patient. Once the steps have been plotted the process starts back at the beginning and evaluates each step in terms of how likely it is to be performed correctly and possible problems that could be encountered at each step. Specifically ask:

- What steps are key to success and maintaining safety?
- How can you encourage that these steps will be made?
- When—at what time points—do distractions occur?
- When are attentions split?
- What steps tend to go wrong, why do they go wrong, and how do they go wrong? (It is important to look at latent root causes and not merely add steps to lessen the likelihood that an individual will make an error as this only adds a burden to the task and is detrimental to the process.)
- How can the chances of these steps going wrong be reduced?

Attention should be paid to log jams, areas where activity and workload is condensed:

- Are there protocols in place that no longer function? Redundant steps that divert attention and are no longer required, merely performed because they always have been?
- Is there any way of spreading this burden out?
- Are necessary steps performed at inappropriate times? Is there a better place for them to be moved to?

Particular attention must be given to areas where information is required to be passed on to new members of the team. For example, at the beginning of anesthesia or at recovery the technician or nurse involved with caring for that patient may know very little about the case:

- How is information passed from team member to team member (information can get lost or distorted if it is passed only by word of mouth)?
- How can information transfer and communication be promoted and encouraged?
- Is there a time when briefing and debriefing about a case can be performed (especially important in a teaching hospital as these time points allow students to reflect on the case and their role in it)?
- Are there verbal and written instructions?
- Can this information and these instructions be presented in a more systematic and repeatable fashion?
- Does the paperwork associated with these time points fulfill its function? Is all relevant information recorded consistently? For example, do you continually get calls asking when a drug should start or what route to give a medication?

In general terms identify how patient information is stored:

- Is there a central store of patient information?
- Is information spread around in different sites?
- Is information available at the kennelside, is it accessible?
- Are the notes always with the patient?
- Is key information about a patient and its condition always available?
- Are forms used in your practice designed properly? Are things being missed? Is it clear whose responsibility it is to complete them?

It is also useful to look not only at the steps themselves but also at the physical environment in which the steps are carried out:

- What is the environment like in which the steps occur?

- Is it cluttered?
- Is everything that is required to safely perform the task readily available?
- Are items stored so they can be found easily?
- Are things labeled well?
- Are items that could be easily confused because of their similarity, stored in the same place?
- Are items used together stored together (e.g., airway devices and airway aids such as laryngoscopes)?
- Are workspaces set out in a logical, linear, and systematic fashion?
- Is there anything that can be feasibly adapted or manipulated to improve steps in the process?
- Can any available tools or equipment be added to help in the performance of each step?
- Is there anything we can remove from the area or relocate that will improve performance?

Conclusion

This chapter has provided some strategies for developing a patient safety mindset, one based on a systems approach that draws upon human factors analysis, as well as tools for managing errors when they occur. Some individuals in veterinary medicine have incorporated these strategies into their day-to-day practice of veterinary anesthesia, but because of the paucity of safety research in veterinary anesthesia, we do not know which strategies are the most practical and effective. The reality is that a single strategy does not exist that will work across the broad spectrum of veterinary anesthesia, but there are fundamental principles that can move us forward.

The imperative first principle is to recognize that we humans make errors; always have and always will. Not intentionally, but this is the reality. Once we acknowledge this, we can be proactive in preventing errors by making them broadly known when they do occur so that all of us can learn from them. This argues for an open and just culture, not only within the practices in which we work, but throughout the broader realm of veterinary anesthesia. We also need to develop the means for recording, analyzing, and reporting error-associated data so that everyone becomes more fully aware of the traps and pitfalls with which we deal on a daily basis. These are fundamental steps that we can and must take.

References

Arriaga, A.F., et al. (2013) Simulation-based trial of surgical-crisis checklists. *New England Journal of Medicine* **368**(3): 246–253.

Berenholtz, S., et al. (2004) Eliminating catheter-related bloodstream infections in the intensive care unit. *Critical Care Medicine* **32**(10): 2014–2020.

Broom, M.A., et al. (2011) Critical phase distractions in anaesthesia and the sterile cockpit concept. *Anaesthesia* **66**(3): 175–179.

Campbell, G., et al. (2012) Distraction and interruption in anaesthetic practice. *British Journal of Anaesthesia* **109**(5): 707–715.

Cook, R.I. & Woods, D.D. (1994) Operating at the sharp end: The complexity of human error. In: *Human Error in Medicine* (ed. M.S. Bogner). Hillsdale, NJ: Lawrence Erlbaum Associates, pp. 255–310.

Croskerry, P. (2003) Cognitive forcing strategies in clinical decision making. *Annals of Emergency Medicine* **41**(1): 110–120.

Croskerry, P., et al. (2013) Cognitive debiasing 1: Origins of bias and theory of debiasing. *BMJ Quality & Safety* **22**(Suppl. 2): ii58–ii64.

Degani, A. & Wiener, E. (1993) Cockpit checklists – concepts, design, and use. *Human Factors* **35**(2): 345–359.

Dekker, S. (2012) *Just Culture: Balancing Safety and Accountability*, 2nd edn. Farnham, Surrey: Ashgate Publishing Ltd.

Fletcher, D.J., et al. (2012) Development and evaluation of a high-fidelity canine patient simulator for veterinary clinical training. *Journal of Veterinary Medical Education* **39**(1): 7–12.

Gagliardi, A.R., et al. (2014) Multiple interacting factors influence adherence, and outcomes associated with surgical safety checklists: A qualitative study. *PloS One* **9**(9): e108585.

Haynes, A.B., et al. (2009) A surgical safety checklist to reduce morbidity and mortality in a global population. *New England Journal of Medicine* **360**(5): 491–499.

Hollnagel, E. (2014) *Safety-I and Safety-II: The Past and Future of Safety Management*. Burlington, VT: Ashgate.

Hubler, M., Koch, T., & Domino, K.B. (eds) (2014) *Complications and Mishaps in Anesthesia*. Berlin: Springer.

Klein, L. (1990) Anesthetic complications in the horse. *Veterinary Clinics of North America Equine Practice* **6**(3): 665–692.

Klemola, U.M. (2000) The psychology of human error revisited. *European Journal of Anaesthesiology* **17**(6): 401.

Klemola, U. & Norros, L. (1997) Analysis of the clinical behaviour of anaesthetists: Recognition of uncertainty as a basis for practice. *Medical Education* **31**(6): 449–456.

Klemola, U. & Norros, L. (2001) Practice-based criteria for assessing anaesthetists' habits of action: Outline for a reflexive turn in practice. *Medical Education* **35**: 455–464.

Leape, L.L. (2014) The checklist conundrum. *New England Journal of Medicine* **370**(11): 1063–1064.

Michie, S., *et al.* (2005) Making psychological theory useful for implementing evidence based practice: A consensus approach. *Quality & Safety in Health Care* **14**(1): 26–33.

Nagano, H. (1975) Report of Japan Air Lines (JAL) Human Factors Working Group. In: *Proceedings of the International Air Transport Association (IATA) Twentieth Technical Conference*. IATA.

Naganobu, K., *et al.* (2001) Arrhythmogenic effect of hypercapnia in ducks anesthetized with halothane. *American Journal of Veterinary Research* **62**(1): 127–129.

Nagpal, K., *et al.* (2010) A systematic quantitative assessment of risks associated with poor communication in surgical care. *Archives of Surgery (Chicago, Ill.: 1960)* **145**(6): 582–588.

Norros, L. & Klemola, U. (1999) Methodological considerations in analysing anaesthetists' habits of action in clinical situations. *Ergonomics* **42**(11): 1521–1530.

Patterson, E.S. & Woods, D. (2001) Shift changes, updates, and the on-call architecture in space shuttle mission control. *Computer Supported Cooperative Work (CSCW)* **10**(3–4): 317–346.

Patterson, E.S., *et al.* (2004) Handoff strategies in settings with high consequences for failure: Lessons for health care operations. *International Journal for Quality in Health Care* **16**(2): 125–132.

Pronovost, P.J., *et al.* (2006) An intervention to decrease catheter-related bloodstream infections in the ICU. *New England Journal of Medicine* **355**(26): 2725–2732.

Reason, J.T. (1990) *Human Error.* Cambridge: Cambridge University Press.

Reason, J.T. (2000) Safety paradoxes and safety culture. *Injury Control and Safety Promotion* **7**(1): 3–14.

Reason, J.T. (2004) Beyond the organisational accident: The need for "error wisdom" on the frontline. *Quality and Safety in Health Care* **13**(Suppl. 2): ii28–ii33.

Roberts, K.H., *et al.* (2005) A case of the birth and death of a high reliability healthcare organisation. *Quality and Safety in Health Care* **14**(3): 216–220.

Ruffato, M., *et al.* (2015) What is the definition of intraoperative hypotension in dogs? Results from a survey of diplomates of the ACVAA and ECVAA. *Veterinary Anaesthesia and Analgesia* **42**(1): 55–64.

Runciman, W.B. & Merry, A.F. (2005) Crises in clinical care: An approach to management. *Quality & Safety in Health Care* **14**(3): 156–163.

Runciman, W.B., *et al.* (1993) Errors, incidents and accidents in anaesthetic practice. *Anaesthesia and Intensive Care* **21**(5): 506–519.

Runciman, W.B., *et al.* (2005) Crisis management during anaesthesia: The development of an anaesthetic crisis management manual. *Quality and Safety in Health Care* **14**(3): e1–e12.

Russ, S., *et al.* (2013) Do safety checklists improve teamwork and communication in the operating room? A systematic review. *Annals of Surgery* **258**(6): 856–871.

Safe Surgery Saves Lives Programme Team (2009) *WHO Guidelines for Safe Surgery 2009: Safe Surgery Saves Lives.* Geneva: World Health Organization.

Stiegler, M.P. & Ruskin, K.J. (2012) Decision-making and safety in anesthesiology. *Current Opinion in Anaesthesiology* **25**(6): 724–729.

Stiegler, M.P. & Tung, A. (2014) Cognitive processes in anesthesiology decision making. *Anesthesiology* **120**(1): 204–217.

Thomassen, O., *et al.* (2014) The effects of safety checklists in medicine: A systematic review. *Acta Anaesthesiologica Scandinavica* **58**(1): 5–18.

Treadwell, J.R., *et al.* (2014) Surgical checklists: A systematic review of impacts and implementation. *BMJ Quality & Safety* **23**(4): 299–318.

Urbach, D.R., *et al.* (2014) Introduction of surgical safety checklists in Ontario, Canada. *New England Journal of Medicine* **370**(11): 1029–1038.

Vogus, T.J. & Hilligoss, B. (2015) The underappreciated role of habit in highly reliable healthcare. *BMJ Quality & Safety* doi:10.1136/bmjqs-2015-004512.

Weed, L.L. (1968) Medical records that guide and teach. *New England Journal of Medicine* **278**(11): 593–600.

Weiser, T.G., *et al.* (2010) Effect of a 19-item surgical safety checklist during urgent operations in a global patient population. *Annals of Surgery* **251**(5): 976–980.

Suggested Readings

The following is a list of suggested readings that relate to errors and accidents. This is not an exhaustive list, but includes texts that have informed and guided us in our thinking about errors.

James Reason. *Human Error.* **Cambridge, UK: Cambridge University Press, 1990.**
Professor James Reason and the study of errors and accidents are synonymous. His research in this field spans over 30 years and this book reflects what he has learned about how and why errors and accidents occur. This text is a must read as it presents a general overall view of the topic, a view that is applicable to a broad range of professional endeavors.

James Reason. *The Human Contribution: Unsafe Acts, Accidents and Heroic Recoveries.* **Farnham, UK: Ashgate Publishing Co., 2008.**
This text explores the human contribution to errors and accidents, but with a few interesting twists. Professor Reason's interest in human actions that have literally "pulled the fat out of the fire" is discussed in depth in this text. In an effort to determine what human characteristics helped individuals avoid catastrophe, he has gone back in time to such historical events as the 1811 retreat of the Light Division at Fuentes de Onoro, and the 1950 withdrawal of the 1st Marine Division from Chosin Reservoir during the Korean War. In presenting these two cases he explores the role of training, discipline, and leadership as crucial factors in overcoming errors and the accidents they can cause. In the chapter on "Sheer Unadulterated Professionalism" he recounts the incredible stories surrounding more contemporary events such as Apollo 13, British Airways Flight 09, United Flight 232, and the Gimli Glider. These stories are riveting in their telling and his analyses of the roles of the key players in these events that saved many lives,

are most informative. This text also reflects Dr Reason's thinking about the balance that needs to be struck between the systems approach to error prevention and resolution and the people approach. He is a proponent of the systems approach, but states that people are the causes of most errors and accidents. For this reason we need to consider how to encourage people at the "sharp edge" to be more proactive in preventing errors and accidents. As he acknowledges, this gets to the essence of Karl Weick's concept of "mindfulness."

David M. Gaba, Kevin J. Fish, & Steven K. Howard. *Crisis Management in Anesthesiology.* **Philadelphia, PA: Churchill Livingstone, 1994.**
An excellent text that specifically discusses errors and accidents in anesthesia. The first two chapters present the theory of dynamic decision-making and crisis resource management. The remainder of the text presents a catalogue of critical events with suggestions as to how they should be managed so as to avoid errors and accidents.

Catherine Marcucci, Norman A. Cohen, David G. Metro, & Jeffrey R. Kirsch (eds) *Avoiding Common Anesthesia Errors.* **Philadelphia, PA: Lippincott Williams & Wilkins, 2008.**
In the Preface the editors write that it had been suggested to them that this text might be titled "Conversations from the Anesthesiology Break Room." This reflects a reality that it is often in the telling of stories within the break room over a cup of coffee that we learn of others' errors, and from them we learn of the traps and pitfalls that can lead so easily to unintended acts. It is a collection of many short sections within broader topics, such as the airway and ventilation, lines and access, medications and equipment, to name only a few. There are some gems in this text; it is easy and enjoyable reading.

Errors in Veterinary Anesthesia, First Edition. John W. Ludders and Matthew McMillan.
© 2017 John Wiley & Sons, Inc. Published 2017 by John Wiley & Sons, Inc.

Sidney Dekker. *The Field Guide to Understanding Human Error.* **Aldershot, UK: Ashgate Publishing Co., 2006.**

The author has extensive experience in flight safety and brings this experience and knowledge to bear in this text, which very much reflects his approach to error prevention, that of the systems approach. It is a general text dealing with error, not specifically in anesthesia. It is as the title suggests, a field guide to understanding and dealing with errors. It is well worth reading.

Sidney Dekker. *Safety Differently: Human Factors for a New Era,* **2nd edition. Boca Raton, FL: CRC Press, 2013.**

A fascinating but frustrating in-depth discussion of how error analysis has evolved and the difficulty in applying human factors analysis to determine how errors occur. It takes as its premise that the human factor should not be viewed as a problem to be controlled, but as a solution to harness, one that sees people as the source of diversity, insight, creativity, and wisdom about safety, not as the source of risk that undermines an otherwise safe system. It discusses in depth the problem of teasing out the many human factors that may be involved in error generation, but does so by discussing how outsiders' biases, especially hindsight bias, may cloud analysis and only identify what the outsider expects to see rather than what the person at the "sharp end" actually experienced. A shortcoming of the book, what makes it frustrating, is that it leaves the reader somewhat adrift as to how to get away from what Dekker calls the Cartesian-Newtonian approach to error analysis that leads us to explain and think about human action in terms of linear sequence(s) of causes and effects.

Atul Gawande. *The Checklist Manifesto.* **Metropolitan Books of Henry Holt and Company LLC, 2009.**

This book explains the evolution of the World Health Organization's Surgical Safety Checklist from its conception to its implementation. Includes insights into the use of checklists in aviation and the building of skyscrapers as well as in medicine. It contains a number of thought-provoking narratives and stories as well as a description of the processes that went into the development of the Surgical Safety Checklist.

Pat Croskerry. Diagnostic failure: A cognitive and affective approach. In: *Advances in Patient Safety: From Research to Implementation. Volume 2: Concepts and Methodology* **(eds Kerm Henriksen, James B. Battles, Eric S. Marks, and David I. Lewin). Rockville, MD: Agency for Healthcare Research and Quality, 2005.**

Gives a good overview of the cognitive and affective states that influence the diagnostic and decision-making process and the conditions that lead to them. It does not outline all possible cognitive biases but does provide an outline of strategies that can help overcome them (debiasing strategies) and how they can be investigated (the cognitive "autopsy").

APPENDIX B

Terminology

The following is a list of terms and their definitions that has been modified from the World Health Organization's (WHO) 2009 report *Conceptual Framework for the International Classification for Patient Safety*. We believe these terms are applicable across the spectrum of veterinary medicine, not just anesthesia. An online source for terminology is PSNet (Patient Safety Network): https:// psnet.ahrq.gov/glossary.

Primary terms

Accountable: being held responsible.

Actions taken to reduce risk: actions taken to reduce, manage, or control any future harm, or probability of harm, associated with an incident.

Adverse incident: an event that caused harm to a patient.

Adverse reaction: unexpected harm resulting from a justified action where the correct process was followed for the context in which the incident occurred.

Ameliorating action: an action taken or circumstances altered to make better or compensate for any harm after an incident has occurred.

Contributing factor: a circumstance, action, or influence that is thought to have played a part in the origin or development of an incident or increased the risk of an incident. Contributing factors include:
Environmental factors
Organizational factors
Human factors
Patient factors
Drug, equipment, or documentation factors

Degree of harm: the severity and duration of harm, and any treatment implications, that result(s) from an incident.

Detection: an action or circumstance that results in the discovery of an incident.

Error: failure to carry out a planned action as intended (error of execution), or use of an incorrect or inappropriate plan (error of planning).

Harmful incident: an incident that reached a patient and caused harm.

Harmless incident: an incident that reached a patient, but did not result in discernible harm.

Hazard: a circumstance, agent, or action with the potential to cause harm.
Agent: a substance, object, or system that acts to produce change.
Circumstance: a situation or factor that may influence an incident, agent, or person(s).

Health: a state of complete physical, mental, and social well-being and not merely the absence of disease or infirmity.

Incident characteristics: selected attributes (qualities, properties, or features) of an incident.

Incident type: a descriptive term for a category consisting of incidents of a common nature, grouped because of shared, agreed features. Incident types consist of:
Behavior
Blood and blood products
Clinical administration
Clinical process or procedure
Communication including documentation
Infrastructure including physical building or fixtures
Medical device or equipment
Medications (any) and includes IV fluids
Nutrition
Oxygen, gas, or vapor
Patient accident (e.g., patient slips and falls, patient breaks tooth on cage bars, patient falls off exam table or transport gurney)

Errors in Veterinary Anesthesia, First Edition. John W. Ludders and Matthew McMillan.
© 2017 John Wiley & Sons, Inc. Published 2017 by John Wiley & Sons, Inc.

Resources or organizational management
Veterinary healthcare-associated infection

Mitigating factor: an action or circumstance that prevents or moderates the progression of an incident toward harming a patient.

Near miss: an incident that for whatever reason, including by chance or timely intervention, did not reach the patient.

Organizational outcome: the impact upon an organization that is wholly or partially attributable to an incident.

Patient characteristics: selected attributes (qualities, properties, or features, including signalment) of a patient.

Patient outcome: the impact upon a patient that is wholly or partially attributable to an incident.

Patient safety: the reduction of risk of unnecessary harm associated with healthcare to an acceptable minimum.

Patient safety incident: a healthcare-related incident or circumstance (situation or factor) that could have resulted, or did result, in unnecessary harm to a patient even if there is no permanent effect on the patient (see "Reportable circumstance").

Preventable: accepted by general consensus as avoidable under the particular set of circumstances.

Quality: the degree to which health services for individuals and populations increase the likelihood of desired health outcomes and are consistent with current professional knowledge.

Reportable circumstance: any situation or factor that could have or did result in unnecessary harm to a patient (see "Patient safety incident").

Resilience: the degree to which a system continuously prevents, detects, mitigates, or ameliorates hazards or incidents.

Risk: the probability that an incident will occur.

Root cause analysis: a systematic iterative process whereby the factors that contribute to an incident are identified by reconstructing the sequence of events and repeatedly asking 'why?' until the underlying root causes have been elucidated.

Safety: the reduction of risk of unnecessary harm to an acceptable minimum.

Side effect: a known effect, other than that primarily intended, related to the pharmacological properties of a medication.

System failure: a fault, breakdown or dysfunction within an organization or practice's operational methods, processes, or infrastructure.

System improvement: the result or outcome of the culture, processes, and structures that are directed toward the prevention of system failure and the improvement of safety and quality.

Veterinary healthcare: services given to an animal or group of animals to promote, maintain, monitor, or restore health.

Veterinary healthcare-associated harm: impairment of structure or function of the body due to plans or actions taken during the provision of healthcare, rather than as a result of an underlying disease or injury; includes disease, injury, suffering, disability, and death:

Disease: any physiological dysfunction.

Injury: damage to tissues caused by an agent or incident.

Suffering: the experience of anything subjectively unpleasant.

Disability: any type of impairment of body structure or function, limitation of activity, or restriction of participation in society, associated with past or present harm.

Veterinary patient: an animal that is a recipient of veterinary healthcare.

Violation: deliberate deviation from an operating procedure, standard, or rule.

Secondary terms

Secondary relevant terms that may be used to further identify or clarify causal factors involved in a patient safety incident.

Active error: an error that occurs at the level of the frontline operator, the effects of which are felt almost immediately.

Active failure: unsafe act committed by people who are in direct contact with the patient or the system and that has an immediate adverse impact on safety by breaching, bypassing, or disabling existing defenses.

Error of commission: an error that occurs as a result of an action taken. For example, administering a drug at the wrong time, in the wrong dosage, or using the wrong route; surgeries performed on the wrong side of the body.

Error of omission: an error that occurs as a result of an action not taken. Errors of omission may or may not lead to an adverse incident.

Fixation bias: persistent failure to revise a diagnosis or plan in the face of readily available evidence that suggests a revision is necessary.

Forcing functions: something that prevents an action from continuing until the problem has been corrected.

Hindsight bias: tendency to view favorably or unfavorably those decisions that have already been made once the outcome is known.

Lapses: internal events that generally involve failures of memory.

Latent conditions: those conditions that exist within a system or organization as a result of design, organizational attributes, training, or maintenance, and that lead to agent errors. These conditions often lie dormant in a system for lengthy periods of time before an incident occurs.

Mistakes: occur when a plan is inadequate to achieve its desired goal even though the actions may be appropriate and run according to plan; mistakes occur at the planning stage of both rule-based and knowledge-based levels of performance.

Negligence: failure to use such care as a reasonably prudent and careful person would under similar circumstances.

Proximate cause: the superficial or obvious act or omission that naturally and directly resulted in an incident. Treating only the proximate cause may lead to short-term improvements, but will not prevent the incident from recurring in a similar or altered form.

Rule-based behavior: decision-making based on familiar rules.

Skill-based behavior: routine tasks requiring little or no conscious attention during execution.

Slip: an error in which the intended action was correct, but the actual action was wrong.

APPENDIX C

ACVAA Monitoring Guidelines

Position Statement (updated 2009)[1]

The American College of Veterinary Anesthesia and Analgesia (ACVAA) has revised the set of guidelines for anesthetic monitoring that were originally developed in 1994 and published in the *Journal of the American Veterinary Medical Association* in 1995 (*JAVMA*, 1995, 206(7): 936–937). Since then many factors have caused a shift in the benchmark used to measure a successful anesthetic outcome, moving from the lack of anesthetic mortality toward decreased anesthetic morbidity.

This shift toward minimizing anesthetic morbidity has been facilitated by more objective definition and earlier detection of pathophysiologic conditions such as hypotension, hypoxemia, and severe hypercapnia. This has resulted from the incorporation of newer monitoring modalities by skilled attentive personnel during anesthesia.

The ACVAA recognizes that it is possible to adequately monitor and manage anesthetized patients without specialized equipment and that some of these modalities may be impractical in certain clinical settings. Furthermore, the ACVAA does not suggest that using any or all the modalities will ensure any specific patient outcome, or that failure to use them will result in poor outcome.

However, as the standard of veterinary care advances and client expectations expand, revised guidelines are necessary to reflect the importance of vigilant monitoring. The goal of the ACVAA guidelines is to improve the level of anesthesia care for veterinary patients. Frequent and continuous monitoring and recording of vital signs in the peri-anesthetic period by trained personnel and the intelligent use of various monitors are requirements for advancing the quality of anesthesia care of veterinary patients.

Circulation

Objective: to ensure adequate circulatory function.

Methods:

1 Palpation of peripheral pulse to determine rate, rhythm, and quality, and evaluation of mucous membrane (MM) color and capillary refill time (CRT).

2 Auscultation of heart beat (stethoscope; esophageal stethoscope, or other audible heart monitor). Continuous (audible heart or pulse monitor) or intermittent monitoring of the heart rate and rhythm.

3 Pulse oximetry to determine the % hemoglobin saturation with oxygen.

4 Electrocardiogram (ECG) continuous display for detection of arrhythmias.

5 Blood pressure:

  a Non-invasive (indirect): oscillometric method: Doppler ultrasonic flow detector.

  b Invasive (direct): arterial catheter connected to an aneroid manometer or to a transducer and oscilloscope.

Recommendations: Continuous awareness of heart rate and rhythm during anesthesia, along with gross assessment of peripheral perfusion (pulse quality, MM color, and CRT) are mandatory. Arterial blood pressure and ECG should also be monitored. There may be some situations where these may be temporarily impractical, e.g., movement of an anesthetized patient to a different area of the hospital.

Oxygenation

Objective: to ensure adequate oxygenation of the patient's arterial blood.

---

[1] Reprinted with permission of the Board of Directors, American College of Veterinary Anesthesia and Analgesia.

Errors in Veterinary Anesthesia, First Edition. John W. Ludders and Matthew McMillan.
© 2017 John Wiley & Sons, Inc. Published 2017 by John Wiley & Sons, Inc.

Methods:

1 Pulse oximetry (non-invasive estimation of hemo-globin saturation).

2 Arterial blood gas analysis for oxygen partial pressure (P_aO_2).

Recommendations: Assessment of oxygenation should be done whenever possible by pulse oximetry, with blood gas analysis being employed when necessary for more critically ill patients.

Ventilation

Objective: to ensure that the patient's ventilation is adequately maintained.

Methods:

1 Observation of thoracic wall movement or observation of breathing bag movement when thoracic wall movement cannot be assessed.

2 Auscultation of breath sounds with an external stethoscope, an esophageal stethoscope, or an audible respiratory monitor.

3 Capnography (end-expired CO_2 measurement).

4 Arterial blood gas analysis for carbon dioxide partial pressure (P_aCO_2).

5 Respirometry (tidal volume measurement).

Recommendations: Qualitative assessment of ventilation is essential as outlined in either 1 or 2 above, and capnography is recommended, with blood gas analysis as necessary.

Temperature

Objective: to ensure that patients do not encounter serious deviations from normal body temperature.

Methods:

1 Rectal thermometer for intermittent measurement.

2 Rectal or esophageal temperature probe for continuous measurement.

Recommendations: Temperature should be measured periodically during anesthesia and recovery, and if possible checked within a few hours after return to the wards.

Neuromuscular blockade

Objective: to assess the intensity of and recovery from neuromuscular blockade.

Methods:

1 Hand-held peripheral nerve stimulator.

2 Spirometer.

Recommendations: For any patient in which neuromuscular blockade is used, it is essential to control ventilation, monitor closely for signs of awareness, and be certain of recovery of blockade prior to anesthesia recovery. Recovery of neuromuscular function may be assumed if the evoked response (twitch and/or tetanic fade) to a nerve stimulus, and respiratory tidal volume as measured with a spirometer, return to at least 70% of pre-blockade status. End-tidal CO_2 may also be used as an indication of adequate ventilation in spontaneously ventilating patients.

Record keeping

Objectives:

1 To maintain a legal record of significant events related to the anesthetic period.

2 To enhance recognition of significant trends or unusual values for physiologic parameters and allow assessment of the response to intervention.

Recommendations:

1 Record all drugs administered to each patient in the peri-anesthetic period and in early recovery, noting the dose, time, and route of administration, as well as any adverse reaction to a drug or drug combination.

2 Record monitored variables on a regular basis (minimum every 5 to 10 minutes) during anesthesia. The minimum variables that should be recorded are heart rate and respiratory rate, as well as oxygenation status and blood pressure if these were monitored.

3 Record heart rate, respiratory rate, and temperature in the early recovery phase.

4 Any untoward events or unusual circumstances should be recorded for legal reasons, and for reference should the patient require anesthesia in the future.

Recovery period

Objective: to ensure a safe and comfortable recovery from anesthesia.

Methods:

1 Observation of respiratory pattern.

2 Observation of mucous membrane color and CRT.

3 Palpation of pulse rate and quality.

4 Measurement of body temperature, with appropriate warming or cooling methods applied if indicated.

5 Observation of any behavior that indicates pain, with appropriate pharmaceutical intervention as necessary.

6 Other measurements as indicated by patient's medical status, e.g., blood glucose, pulse oximetry, PCV, TP, blood gases, etc.

Recommendations: Monitoring in recovery should include at the minimum evaluation of pulse rate and quality, mucous membrane color, respiratory pattern, signs of pain, and temperature.

Personnel

Objective: to ensure that a responsible individual is aware of the patient's status at all times during anesthesia and recovery, and is prepared either to intervene when indicated, or to alert the veterinarian in charge about changes in the patient's condition.

Recommendations:

1 Ideally, a veterinarian, technician, or other responsible person should remain with the patient continuously and be dedicated to that patient only

2 If this is not possible, a reliable and knowledgeable person should check the patient's status on a regular basis (at least every 5 minutes) during anesthesia and recovery.

3 A responsible person may be present in the same room, although not necessarily solely occupied with the anesthetized patient (for instance, the surgeon may also be responsible for overseeing anesthesia).

4 In either of (2) or (3) above, audible heart and respiratory monitors must be available.

5 A responsible person, solely dedicated to managing and caring for the anesthetized patient during anesthesia, remains with the patient continuously until the end of the anesthetic period (a, b):

a Recommended for all patients assessed as ASA status III, IV, or V.

b Recommended for horses anesthetized with inhalation anesthetics and/or horses anesthetized for longer than 45 minutes.

Sedation without general anesthesia

Sedation is a state characterized by central depression accompanied by drowsiness during which the patient is generally unaware of its surroundings but responsive to noxious manipulation [Thurmon JC, Short CE (2007) History and Overview of Veterinary Anesthesia. In: *Lumb & Jones' Veterinary Anesthesia and Analgesia* (4th Edition), Tranquilli WJ, Thurmon JC, Grimm KA (eds). Blackwell Publishing, Ames, Iowa, p. 5]. If a sedated patient is sufficiently obtunded to lose control of protective airway reflexes, it should be monitored as under general anesthesia.

Objective: to ensure adequate oxygenation and hemodynamic stability in the obtunded patient.

Methods:

1 Palpation of pulse rate, rhythm, and quality.

2 Observation of mucous membrane color and CRT.

3 Observation of respiratory rate and pattern.

4 Auscultation.

5 Pulse oximetry.

6 Oxygen supplementation.

Recommendation: Intermittent monitoring of basic respiratory and cardiovascular parameters in the heavily sedated animal should be routine. Supplemental oxygen, an endotracheal tube, and materials for IV catheterization should always be readily available. Particular attention should be paid to brachycephalic breeds, which are particularly at risk for airway obstruction under heavy sedation

ACVAA Guidelines for Anesthesia in Horses[1]

Prepared by the ACVA Equine Standards Committee: Elizabeth A. Martinez, Ann E. Wagner, Bernd Driessen, Cynthia Trim.

I Preoperative Evaluation

  A History

  1 Response to prior sedation or anesthesia

  2 History of any significant illness or injury

  3 Current problem

  B Physical Examination

  1 Temperature, pulse rate, respiratory rate

  2 Evaluation of all organ systems, focusing on the presence or absence of cardiovascular and respiratory abnormalities

  3 Capillary refill time, mucous membrane color

  C Laboratory Blood Work

  1 Order or perform any necessary blood work.

  2 Recommended tests, if any, will depend on physical status of the patient and the procedure to be performed.

II Selection of Anesthetic Regimen

  A An appropriate regimen should be chosen based on:

  1 Physical status of patient

  2 Duration of anesthesia required

  3 Number and skill of personnel available

  4 Safety of facility or location where anesthesia (including induction and recovery) will be performed

  5 Anesthetic equipment available

  6 Monitoring equipment available

  B Total Intravenous Anesthesia (TIVA)

  1 Recommended for procedures expected to be 1 hour or less in duration

  2 Muscle relaxation may not be as profound compared to inhalant anesthesia

  3 Anesthetic agents may be administered as intermittent boluses or as an intravenous infusion

  C Inhalant Anesthesia

  1 Preferred for lengthy procedures (>1 hour of anesthesia time)

  2 Requires additional equipment compared to TIVA

  3 Commonly used inhalants include halothane, isoflurane, sevoflurane

III Monitoring and Supportive Care

  A Intravenous catheterization is recommended for administration of anesthetic drugs, fluids, and supportive medications

  B Proper position and padding is vital to aid in prevention of muscle or nerve injury

  C TIVA

  1 Oxygen source+flowmeter for nasal insufflation, if indicated

  2 Endotracheal tubes and demand valve readily available to ventilate, if necessary

  3 Pad/cloth for face and eye

  D Inhalant Anesthesia

  1 Appropriately sized, cuffed, endotracheal tube

  2 Oxygen source+anesthesia machine

  3 Means to scavenge anesthetic waste gases

  4 Means to manually or mechanically ventilate, if necessary

  E Monitoring of the cardiovascular system

  1 Digital pulse palpation

  2 CRT, mucous membrane color

  3 ECG, if indicated

  4 Arterial blood pressure, if indicated (strongly recommended whenever inhalation anesthesia is used)

  5 Hypotension should be treated with appropriate medication (fluids, inotropes, etc.)

---

[1]Reprinted with permission of the Board of Directors, American College of Veterinary Anesthesia and Analgesia.

Errors in Veterinary Anesthesia, First Edition. John W. Ludders and Matthew McMillan.
© 2017 John Wiley & Sons, Inc. Published 2017 by John Wiley & Sons, Inc.

F Monitoring of the respiratory system
  1 Observation of respiratory rate and rhythm
  2 Pulse oximetry, if indicated
  3 Capnometry, if indicated (note: ETCO$_2$ frequently underestimates P_aCO_2 in anesthetized horses)
  4 Arterial blood gas analysis, if indicated
  5 Hypoventilation is treated with either assisted or controlled ventilation

IV Injectable adjuncts during anesthesia
  A May be useful to provide additional anesthesia, analgesia, or muscle relaxation during anesthesia.
  B May be administered as a bolus or, with certain medications, be given as a constant rate infusion.
  C Common adjuncts include:
    1 Opioids (e.g., butorphanol)
    2 Ketamine
    3 Local anesthetics (either intravenously or as a local or regional technique)
    4 Muscle relaxants
      a Diazepam or midazolam
      b Guaifenesin
      c Neuromuscular blocking agents (controlled ventilation and monitoring of neuromuscular function is required during paralysis)

V Local and regional analgesia/anesthesia
  A May be chosen as the sole technique for certain procedures.
  B Depending on the temperament of the patient and type of procedure, chemical restraint may also be used in combination with a local or regional technique.
  C May also be used as an adjunct to general anesthesia.

D Choice of local anesthetics includes lidocaine, mepivacaine, and bupivacaine. The addition of epinephrine (5 micrograms/mL) may help to improve the quality and duration of anesthesia.
E Local and regional techniques include:
  1 Local infiltration (e.g., line block, ring block)
  2 Peripheral nerve block
  3 Intra-articular block
  4 Paravertebral block
  5 Epidural analgesia/anesthesia
    a Local anesthetics
    b Alpha-2 agonists

VI Recovery
  A TIVA
    1 If in padded, confined area (recovery stall), no assistance may be needed
    2 If in open area (outside), area should be relatively soft (grass), free of obstacles (trees, fences, stakes, rocks), and assistance should be provided to prevent too much momentum
      a Control head, protect eyes
      b Assist on tail (if possible)
  B Inhalant Anesthesia
    1 Depending on temperament and physical status of horse, inhalant used, surgical procedure performed, and design of recovery stall, the horse may recover either unassisted or with assistance on the head and/or tail.
    2 If recovery is unassisted, the patient should be observed as often as needed to be able to identify if the horse unexpectedly requires assistance.
    3 Sedatives and/or analgesics may be administered during the recovery period to aid in a smooth transition to standing.

APPENDIX E

A Brief History of Checklists

As discussed throughout this book, anesthesia is often compared to flying an aircraft, with key processes being takeoff (induction) and landing (recovery) with only occasional issues occurring during flight (maintenance). Aviation has taught us a lot about error and human factors and it has also introduced a number of novel solutions. One of the most important of these is the humble checklist.

Like many advances in medicine, the safety checklist has its history rooted in the military. In 1935 the US Army Air Corps started a final set of aircraft evaluations at Wright Field, Dayton, Ohio. On the line was a contract to supply the US Army with potentially up to 200 long-range bomber aircraft.

There were three aircraft competing for this large and lucrative contract, one of which was the Boeing Model 299. Legend has it that all initial evaluations (consisting of about 40 hours of flight time) had gone in Boeing's favor and the final flight was a mere formality. Boeing's entry had already earned itself the nickname "the Flying Fortress," as it could carry considerably more bombs and fly faster and farther than the other two entries. Flying the Model 299 that day were two highly experienced Army pilots, Boeing's chief test pilot, along with a Boeing mechanic and a representative of the engine manufacturer. After takeoff the Model 299 began to climb but within a few seconds the aircraft stalled and fell to the ground, bursting into flames upon impact. Although all onboard escaped or were rescued, both pilots later died of their injuries.

Compared to a typical plane at the time, the Model 299 was a complex aircraft with additional controls and instruments that required attention. Finding no evidence of mechanical malfunction the accident investigation team assigned to the crash concluded that "pilot error" was the cause. Evidently the pilots had made a simple but fatal mistake with one of the new controls, leaving the elevator and rudder controls locked. A newspaper at the time went on to state that the Model 299 was just "too much plane for one man to fly."

This could have been the end of the story but for the huge potential advantage the bomber would give the US army if it could be flown safely. So although the main contract was for the Douglass DB-1, a dozen Model 299 planes were purchased for testing purposes. After some deliberation the solution to the problem was simple, ingenious, but most of all effective: the pilots' checklist. It turned out the plane was not too much for one man, but merely too much for one man's memory; a simple checklist could ensure that none of the crucial steps during the key periods of flight were forgotten.

Four checklists were initially developed: takeoff, flight, before landing, and after landing. All pilots were taught how to use the checklist as part of their normal flight training. The initial 12 Model 299s tested by the army went on to fly almost 2 million miles without serious incident and the army went on to order over ten thousand. The army renamed the aircraft B-17 and it became an icon, a symbol of power for the US Air Force.

The checklist idea was so successful that it enabled aviation and aeronautical engineering to become more and more complex. Checklists were developed for more and more parts of flight, for emergency situations as well as more routine situations. As an example, checklists were developed for almost every part of the Apollo missions and all astronauts were trained in how to use them and write them. Each of the Apollo 11 astronauts logged over 100 hours of time familiarizing themselves with and adapting these checklists. In fact, checklists were so integral to the success of the Apollo moon landings that astronaut Michael Collins coined them "The fourth crew member."

Errors in Veterinary Anesthesia, First Edition. John W. Ludders and Matthew McMillan.
© 2017 John Wiley & Sons, Inc. Published 2017 by John Wiley & Sons, Inc.

FDA Anesthesia Apparatus Checkout[1]

This checkout, or a reasonable equivalent, should be conducted before administration of anesthesia. These recommendations are only valid for an anesthesia system that conforms to current and relevant standards and includes an ascending bellows ventilator and at least the following monitors: capnograph, pulse oximeter, oxygen analyzer, respiratory volume monitor (spirometer), and breathing system pressure monitor with high- and low-pressure alarms. This is a guideline that users are encouraged to modify to accommodate differences in equipment design and variations in local clinical practice. Such local modifications should have appropriate peer review. Users should refer to the operator's manual for the manufacturer's specific procedures and precautions, especially the manufacturer's low-pressure leak test (step number V).

Emergency Ventilation Equipment

I ***Verify Backup Ventilation Equipment is Available and Functioning**

High Pressure System

II ***Check O$_2$ Cylinder Supply**

  A Open O$_2$ cylinder and verify at least half full (about 1000 psi).

  B Close cylinder.

III ***Check Central Pipeline Supplies**

  A Check that hoses are connected and pipeline gauges read about 50 psi.

Low Pressure System

IV ***Check Initial Status of Low Pressure System**

  A Close flow control valves and turn vaporizers off.

  B Check fill level and tighten vaporizers' filler caps.

V ***Perform Leak Check of Machine Low Pressure System**

  A Verify that the machine master switch and flow control valves are OFF.

  B Attach "suction bulb" to common fresh gas outlet.

  C Squeeze bulb repeatedly until fully collapsed.

  D Verify bulb stays fully collapsed for at least 10 seconds.

  E Open one vaporizer at a time and repeat C and D as above.

  F Remove suction bulb, and reconnect fresh gas hose.

VI ***Turn On Machine Master Switch and all other necessary electrical equipment**

VII ***Test Flowmeters**

  A Adjust flow of all gases through their full range, checking for smooth operation of floats and undamaged flowtubes.

  B Attempt to create a hypoxic O$_2$/N$_2$O mixture and verify correct changes in flow and/or alarm.

Scavenging System

VIII ***Adjust and Check Scavenging System**

  A Ensure proper connections between the scavenging system and both APL (pop-off) valve and ventilator relief valve.

  B Adjust waste gas vacuum (if possible).

  C Fully open APL valve and occlude Y-piece.

---

[1]From: US Government, Department of Health and Human Services, Food and Drug Administration, 1993.

---

*NOTE: If an anesthetist uses the same machine in successive cases, these steps (*) need not be repeated or may be abbreviated after the initial checkout.

Errors in Veterinary Anesthesia, First Edition. John W. Ludders and Matthew McMillan.
© 2017 John Wiley & Sons, Inc. Published 2017 by John Wiley & Sons, Inc.

D With minimum O_2 flow, allow scavenger reservoir bag to collapse completely and verify that absorber pressure gauge reads about zero.

E With the O_2 flush activated allow the scavenger reservoir bag to distend fully, and then verify that absorber pressure gauge reads <10 cmH_2O.

Breathing System

IX ***Calibrate O_2 Monitor**

A Ensure monitor reads 21% in room air.

B Verify low-oxygen alarm is enabled and functioning.

C Reinstall sensor in circuit and flush breathing system with oxygen.

D Verify that monitor now reads greater than 90%.

X **Check Initial Status of Breathing System**

A Set selector switch to "Bag" mode.

B Check that breathing circuit is complete, undamaged, and unobstructed.

C Verify that CO_2 absorbent is adequate.

D Install breathing circuit accessory equipment (e.g., humidifier, PEEP valve) to be used during the case.

XI **Perform Leak Check of the Breathing System**

A Set all gas flows to zero (or minimum).

B Close APL (pop-off) valve and occlude Y-piece.

C Pressurize breathing system to about 30 cm H_2O with O_2 flush.

D Ensure that pressure remains fixed for at least 10 seconds.

E Open APL (pop-off) valve and ensure that pressure decreases.

Manual and Automatic Ventilation Systems

XII **Test Ventilation Systems and Unidirectional Valves**

A Place a second breathing bag on Y-piece.

B Set appropriate ventilator parameters for next patient.

C Switch to automatic ventilation (Ventilator) mode.

D Fill bellows and breathing bag with O_2 flush and then turn ventilator ON.

E Set O_2 flow to minimum, other gas flows to zero.

F Verify that during inspiration bellows delivers appropriate tidal volume and that during expiration bellows fills completely.

G Set fresh gas flow to about 5 L/min.

H Verify that the ventilator bellows and simulated lungs fill and empty appropriately without sustained pressure at end expiration.

I Check for proper action of unidirectional valves.

J Exercise breathing circuit accessories to ensure proper function.

K Turn ventilator OFF and switch to manual ventilation (Bag/APL) mode.

L Ventilate manually and assure inflation and deflation of artificial lungs and appropriate feel of system resistance and compliance.

M Remove second breathing bag from Y-piece.

Monitors

XIII **Check, Calibrate, and/or Set Alarm Limits of all Monitors**

A Capnometer

B Pulse Oximeter

C Oxygen Analyzer

D Respiratory Volume Monitor (Spirometer)

E Pressure Monitor with High and Low Airway Alarms

Final Position

XIV **Check Final Status of Machine**

A Vaporizers off

B APL valve open

C Selector switch to "Bag"

D All flowmeters to zero

E Patient suction level adequate

F Breathing system ready to use

Association of Veterinary Anaesthetists Anaesthetic Safety Checklist

Pre-Induction

☐ Patient NAME, owner CONSENT & PROCEDURE confirmed

☐ IV CANNULA placed and patent

☐ AIRWAY EQUIPMENT available and functioning

☐ Endotracheal tube CUFFS checked

☐ ANAESTHETIC MACHINE checked today

☐ Adequate OXYGEN for proposed procedure

☐ BREATHING SYSTEM connected, leak free & APL VALVE OPEN

☐ Person assigned to MONITOR patient

☐ Risks identified & COMMUNICATED

☐ EMERGENCY INTERVENTIONS available

Pre-Procedure – Time Out

☐ Patient NAME & PROCEDURE confirmed

☐ DEPTH of anaesthesia appropriate

☐ SAFETY CONCERNS COMMUNICATED

Recovery

☐ SAFETY CONCERNS COMMUNICATED

☐ Airway, Breathing, Circulation (fluid balance), Body Temperature, Pain

☐ ASSESSMENT & INTERVENTION PLAN confirmed

☐ ANALGESIC PLAN confirmed

☐ Person assigned to MONITOR patient

Recommended Procedures

Pre-Anaesthesia

★ Has anything significant been identified in the history and/or clinical examination?

★ Do any abnormalities warrant further investigation?

★ Can any abnormalities be stabilised prior to anaesthesia?

★ What complications are anticipated during anaesthesia?

★ How can these complications be managed?

★ Would the patient benefit from premedication?

★ How will any pain associated with the procedure be managed?

★ How will anaesthesia be induced & maintained?

★ How will the patient be monitored?

★ How will the patient's body temperature be maintained?

★ How will the patient be managed in the post-anaesthetic period?

★ Are the required facilities, personnel & drugs available?

Anaesthetic Machine

☐ PRIMARY OXYGEN source checked

☐ BACK-UP OXYGEN available

☐ OXYGEN ALARM working (if present)

☐ FLOWMETERS working

☐ VAPORIZER attached and working

☐ Anaesthetic machine passes LEAK TEST

☐ SCAVENGING checked

☐ Available MONITORING equipment functioning

☐ EMERGENCY equipment and drugs checked

Drugs/Equipment

• Endotracheal tubes (cuffs checked)

• Airway aids (e.g. laryngoscope, urinary catheter, lidocaine spray, suction, guide-wire/stylet)

• Self-inflating bag (or demand valve for equine anaesthetics)

• Epinephrine/adrenaline

• Atropine

• Antagonists (e.g. atipamezole, naloxone/butorphanol)

• Intravenous cannulae

• Isotonic crystalloid solution

• Fluid administration set

Drug charts & CPR algorithm (http://www.acvecc-recover.org/)

Available at: http://www.ava.eu.com/resources/checklists/
Reproduced with permission of the Association of Veterinary Anaesthetists (AVA).

Critical Clinical Condition Checklists

The following checklists were created for use at the Queen's Veterinary Hospital, University of Cambridge. It is a listing of critical clinical conditions that may be encountered during anesthesia plus considerations for further assessment and interventions. The interventions and drug doses herein are guidelines only based on the author's (M.W.M.) experience, they are not absolutes. An animal's clinical condition will dictate interventions including drugs and doses.

Errors in Veterinary Anesthesia, First Edition. John W. Ludders and Matthew McMillan.
© 2017 John Wiley & Sons, Inc. Published 2017 by John Wiley & Sons, Inc.

HYPOTENSION

- **Description:** Drop in blood pressure (suggested threshold MAP 60 mmHg, SAP 80 mmHg). Inability to obtain NIBP measurements, weak/absent peripheral pulses
- **Objective:** Restore haemodynamic stability

---

1 **If haemorrhage, anaphylaxis, tachycardia or bradycardia see relevant checklists**

2 **VAPORISER SETTING**
   reduce and consider altering anaesthetic protocol (provide supplemental anaesthesia/analgesia)

3 **FLUID BOLUS**
   10–30 mL/kg isotonic crystalloid (LRS or NaCl 0.9%)
   2–5 mL/kg colloid and reassess response
   Respiratory pulse profile variation (esp. following intermittent positive pressure ventilation (IPPV))
      indicates likely fluid responsiveness

4 **PHARMACOLOGICAL SUPPORT**

Inotropes-	Dobutamine 1–10 µg/kg/min
	Dopamine 5–10 µg/kg/min
Vasopressors-	Phenylephrine 2–10 µg/kg q 5–15 min or 0.1–1 µg/kg/min
Mixed vasopressor/intropes-	Ephedrine 50–100 µg/kg q 20 min (max. 3 times)
	Epinephrine 0.1–2 µg/kg/min
	Norepinephrine 0.1–1 µg/kg/min
	Dopamine >10 µg/kg/min

HAEMORRHAGE
- Blood in site
- Blood in suction
- Blood on swabs
- Blood on table/floor/hidden by drapes
- Occult bleeding—history of trauma?

HYPOVOLAEMIA OF OTHER CAUSE
- Large swing in pulse profile following PPV
- History of pre-anaesthetic volume deficit

VASODILATION
- Too deep?
- Acepromazine
- Possibility of SIRS/sepsis
- Vagal stimulation
- Anaphylaxis—bronchoconstriction/urticaria
- Release of vasoactive substances

OBSTRUCTION
- Vascular compression—surgeon
- Mass effect (obesity, pregnancy, organomegaly)

CONTRACTILITY
- Myocardial disease—cardiomyopathy
- Drug related
- Disease related—hypothyroidism, critical illness
- Age—paediatric, geriatric

ARRHYTHMIA
- Bradycardia—"Too slow to flow" (sinus bradycardia, AV block)
- Tachycardia—"Too fast to fill" (VTach, AF, SVT)

OTHER
- Rapid removal of a chronic abdominal effusion
- Ligation of a major vessel—PDA/PSS/renal vein
- Sudden change in body position (e.g. sternal to dorsal)

HAEMORRHAGE

- **Description:** Massive uncontrolled haemorrhage
- **Objective:** Maintain perfusion to major organs whilst minimising haemorrhage and coagulopathy until haemorrhage controlled. Restore haemodynamic stability

---

1 **CONTROL HAEMORRHAGE**
   tourniquet, pressure, clamp, haemostatic dressings

2 **FLUID BOLUSES**
   open IV and bolus isotonic crystalloid (LRS or 0.9% NaCl preferably warmed) 10–30 mL/kg
   repeat as necessary
   1:1 to 2:1 with blood volume lost
   90 mL/kg = blood volume in a dog
   60 mL/kg = blood volume in a cat

3 **FIO2 100%**

4 **REDUCE VAPORISER SETTING**
   reduce and consider altering anaesthetic protocol (provide supplemental anaesthesia/analgesia)

5 **ESTIMATE LOSS**
   weigh swabs, volume in suction, volume on table/floor

6 **BLOOD PRODUCTS**
   transfusion trigger >30% blood loss or PCV <20% or Hb 7 g/dL in dogs (15%, 5 g/dL in cats)
   Fresh whole blood ideal (contains platelets)
   otherwise fresh frozen plasma + packed RBCs 1:1

7 **HYPOTENSIVE RESUSCITATION**
   Consider if unable to control haemorrhage
   Maintain MAP between 50–60 mmHg
   SAP 80–90 mmHg (just palpable peripheral pulses) reduces ongoing blood loss

8 **MAINTAIN NORMOTHERMIA**
   Hypothermia = coagulopathy
   Warm patient, environment, lavage and fluids

9 **COAGULOPATHY**
   Continued oozing at surgical sites
   FFP (10–15 mL/kg)
   Consider cryoprecipitate, tranexamic acid 10 mg/kg

BRADYCARDIA

- **Description:** Sudden decrease in heart rate or heart rate below 60 bpm in dogs and below 80 bpm in cats

- **Objective:** Ensure adequate perfusion. Increase heart rate if required

---

1 **CHECK PRESSURE**

   Is the heart rate affecting perfusion pressure?

   Is heart rate an effect of blood pressure? (baroreceptor reflex)- If yes see **HYPERTENSION** checklist

2 **ECG**

   Can you identify the rhythm?

3 **ELECTROLYTES-**

   Is an electrolyte disturbance likely (K^+ or Ca^{2+})?

   If yes check and correct as required

4 **ANTAGONISE ALPHA-2 AGONISTS**

   Atipamazole for dogs at:

      5 times medetomidine dose (equal volume)

      10 times dexmedetomidine dose (equal volume)

   Atipamazole for cats at:

      2.5 times medetomidine dose (half volume)

      5 times dexmedetomidine dose (half volume)

5 **ANTICHOLINERGICS**

   Atropine 20–50 µg/kg

   Glycopyrrolate 5–10 µg/kg

   May cause reflex bradycardia before heart rate increases

6 **REDUCE VAPORISER SETTING**

   Especially relevant if hypothermic as hypothermia increases depth of anaesthesia

7 **WARM HYPOTHERMIC PATIENTS**

   Warm patient, environment, lavage and fluids

8 **ADRENERGIC AGENTS**

   Useful in hypothermic patients

   Ephedrine 50–100 µg/kg

   Epinephrine 1–10 µg/kg diluted given slowly

VAGALLY MEDIATED
- Pharmacological (Opioids & Alpha-2 agonists)
- Reflex or surgical manipulation (oculo-vagal, trigeminal vagal, neck— vagovagal, baroreceptor, cranial, abdomen, thorax, Bezold–Jarisch reflex)

HYPOTHERMIA
- Any cause (especially with hypovolaemia in cats)

PRIMARY ARRHYTHMIA
- AV block (3rd degree) or sick sinus syndrome

RAISED ICP
- Cushing's reflex (hypertension, bradycardia, respiratory abnormalities)

LOCAL ANAESTHETIC TOXICITY
Potential of overdose if >4 mg/kg lidocaine, 2 mg/kg bupivacaine or IV administration

HYPERKALAEMIA
- Acute kidney injury (AKI)
- Urinary bladder rupture or urethral blockage
- Hypoadrenocorticism (Addison's)
- Cellular- reperfusion injury/massive trauma/haemolysis
- Inadvertent rapid administration of fluids supplemented with KCl

HYPERCALCAEMIA
- Pathophysiological—paraneoplastic, renal, hyperparathyroidism
- Toxicity

TACHYCARDIA

- **Description:** Sudden elevation in heart rate or heart rate above 180 in dogs or above 220 in cats
- **Objective:** Ensure adequate perfusion. Decrease heart rate if required

---

1 **BLOOD PRESSURE**

Is hypovolaemia possible cause?

Is rate affecting cardiac output? Poor pulses?

Hypertension+tachycardia could indicate pain or inadequate depth of anaesthesia or sympathetic storm

2 **PULSE DEFICITS?**

3 **ENSURE DEPTH**

Check and correct if required

4 **ENSURE ANALGESIA**

Opioids—fentanyl 1–5 μg/kg, methadone 0.1 mg/kg (may need IPPV)

5 **ECG**

IF supraventricular tachycardia (SVT) consider:

Opioids—fentanyl 1–5 μg/kg, methadone 0.1 mg/kg (may need IPPV)

Beta-blockers—esmolol 0.05–0.5 mg/kg then 25–200 μg/kg/min

IF Vtach consider:

Lidocaine 2 mg/kg boluses (max. 3) then 50–100 μg/kg/h

Then magnesium 40 mg/kg followed by 15 mg/kg/h, or beta-blockers such as esmolol as above

IF NO ECG:

Check for fluid responsiveness

Opioids as above

Lidocaine as above

6 **ELECTROLYTES**

Is an electrolyte disturbance likely (K^+ or Ca^{2+} or Mg^{2+})?

If yes, check and correct as required

Sympathetic origin
- Baroreceptor reflex (see "Hypotension")
- Pain
- Inadequate depth of anaesthesia
- Hormonal—hyperthyroidism (thyroid storm), primary adrenergic (sympathetic storm—phaeochromocytoma)
- Pharmacological—anticholinergics, beta-agonists
- Hypoxia

Primary cardiac
- Primary arrhythmia—SVT, AFib, Vtach, Arrhythmogenic Right Ventricular Cardiomyopathy (ARVCM)
- Myocardial disease (DCM, HCM, mitral valve disease)
- Myocardial injury

Other
- Vtach due to abdominal/inflammatory disease
- Electrolyte abnormalities (hypokalaemia, Ca^{2+} abnormalities, hypomagnesaemia)

> ### HYPOXAEMIA/Hb OXYGEN DESATURATION
>
> - **Description:** Drop in SpO_2 below 93% or PaO_2 below 60 mmHg or a $PaO_2:F_IO_2$ of <200
> - **Objective:** Restore adequate oxygenation

1 **FIO_2 100%**

2 **HAND VENTILATE**
   Is the chest moving?
   Is resistance/compliance normal?
   Is there a CO_2 trace on the capnograph?

3 **CONFIRM AIRWAY**
   Ensure no blockage (airway secretions, haemorrhage, poorly placed ETT)
   Endobronchial intubation

4 **CHECK OXYGEN SOURCE**
   Oxygen concentrator working (oxygen meter confirming F_IO_2)
   Flowmeters working

5 **CHECK BREATHING SYSTEM**
   Leaks (holes, tears, etc.)
   Disconnection

6 **ENSURE ADEQUATE PERFUSION**
   See "Hypotension" checklist

7 **CONSIDER:**
   Suctioning airway
   Re-intubating
   Changing breathing system
   Reducing depth of anaesthesia
   Salbutamol inhaler
   Recruitment manoeuvre if blood pressure adequate
   Instigating PEEP
   Terminate procedure
   Arterial blood gas analysis

Low F_IO_2
- Oxygen source failed

Hypoventilation
- Post-induction apnoea
- Inappropriate depth
- Cervical spinal disease
- Neuromuscular disease
- Pharmacological (NMBA, opioids, ketamine)
- External—obesity, panting, diaphragmatic splinting, pleural space disease

Diffusion barrier impairment
- Fibrotic lung disease (old terriers esp. WHWT, cats with chronic FAS)

V:Q mismatch
- Oedema—protein-rich (ALI, ARDS, TRALI, inflammatory, neurogenic), protein-free (fluid overload, left-sided heart failure)
- Haemorrhage—pulmonary contusions, coagulopathy
- Atelectasis—prolonged recumbency, diaphragmatic splinting, pleural space disease, obesity, NMBA, prolonged anaesthesia with 100% O_2
- Hypotension
- Airway disease—asthma, bronchial disease
- Other—pus (bronchopneumonia, aspirated fluid)

Shunt
- PDA, PFO, VSD, ASD
- Neoplasia
- Severe pulmonary disease

APNOEA/RESPIRATORY ARREST

- **Description:** Cessation in spontaneous respiration
- **Objective:** Adequately ventilate lungs, restore spontaneous ventilation

---

1 **VENTILATE**

   Administer two positive pressure breaths of 100% O_2

   Airway patent? Visualised? CO_2 trace on the capnograph? Chest moves with intermittent positive pressure ventilation (IPPV)?

   Check for ET tube cuff leak

2 **CHECK PULSES; IF ABSENT START CPR ALGORITHM**

3 **DEPTH**

   IF TOO DEEP—wait

   IF TOO LIGHT—start isoflurane and give two more breaths then reassess

4 **SpO_2**

   Monitor and administer two positive pressure breaths if below 93%

5 **$ETCO_2$**

   Administer two positive pressure breaths per minute allowing $ETCO_2$ to increase up to 50-55 mmHg to stimulate spontaneous respiration

---

ANAPHYLAXIS/ALLERGIC REACTION

- **Description:** Urticaria, vasodilation, bronchoconstriction
- **Objective:** Remove trigger. Reverse bronchospasm and vasodilation. Control immune reaction

---

1 **STOP TRIGGER**

   Stop all potential triggers (antibiotics most common)

2 **FIO2 100%**

If mild:

3 **ANTIHISTAMINES**

   Chlorpheniramine 5–10 mg per dog IM (5 mg per cat)
   Ranitidine 1.5 mg/kg IM

4 **CORTICOSTEROIDS**

   Dexamethasone 0.1–0.5 mg/kg

If severe:

5 **ADRENERGIC AGENTS**

   Epinephrine: 1–10 μg/kg q 1–2 minutes or 0.1–2 μg/kg/min after bolus
   Salbutamol: 1 puff of 100 μg per "puff" for small patients, 2 for medium-sized and 3 for large patients

6 **TERMINATE PROCEDURE?**

HYPERTENSION

- **Description:** Sudden increase in blood pressure, SAP over 160mmHg
- **Objective:** Restore normotension

---

1 **HEART RATE**

Hypertension+tachycardia could indicate pain or inadequate depth of anaesthesia or sympathetic storm

2 **ENSURE DEPTH**

Check and correct if required?
Consider deliberately deepening anaesthesia?

3 **ENSURE ANALGESIA**

Opioids—fentanyl 1–5µg/kg, methadone 0.1mg/kg (may need IPPV)
Lidocaine 1–2mg/kg slow IV
Consider patient body position—esp. old patients with DJD (elbow/hip position)

4 **ANTIHYPERTENSIVES**

Consider acepromazine 10µg/kg
Consider magnesium 40mg/kg then 15mg/kg/h
Consider phentolamine 0.02–0.1µg/kg/min then 1–2µg/kg/min
Consider nitroprusside 0.5–15µg/kg/min

HYPERKALAEMIA - HYPERKALAEMIC MYOCARDIAL TOXICITY

- **Description:** Increase in serum K$^+$ leading to myocardial toxicity and arrhythmia
- **Objective:** Restore myocardial membrane stability and correct hyperkalaemia

---

1 **ECG**

2 **STABILISE MYOCARDIUM**

Where bradycardia and signs of hyperkalaemic toxicity are present use calcium as first-line treatment
Calcium (boro)gluconate 50 mg/kg over 5–20 min
0.5 mL/kg of 10% solution IV
Can repeat 2–3 times
Effects will last approx. 15–20 min

3 **REDUCE POTASSIUM LEVELS**

DILUTION: If patient hypotensive/hypoperfused administer isotonic crystalloids (LRS or 0.9%
   NaCl) as required to restore adequate perfusion
INCREASED UPTAKE:
Salbutamol—1 puff of 100 μg per "puff" for small patients, 2 for medium-sized and 3 for large patients
Soluble insulin—0.5 IU/kg with glucose 1–1.5 g/IU insulin as bolus and glucose 1–1.5 g/IU insulin
   over 4–6 h)—monitor blood glucose
Bicarbonate—0.5–1 mEq/kg over 20–30 min

4 **CORRECT UNDERLYING CAUSE**

Check for urinary obstruction (bladder size?)
Check for acute kidney injury
Check for free urine abdomen/retroperitoneal space

Index

Errors in Veterinary Anesthesia, First Edition. John W. Ludders and Matthew McMillan.
© 2017 John Wiley & Sons, Inc. Published 2017 by John Wiley & Sons, Inc.

Printed and bound by CPI Group (UK) Ltd, Croydon, CR0 4YY

16/04/2025

14658459-0004

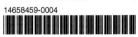